MW00438771

Medical Assisting

Fourth Edition

Lippincott Williams & Wilkins'

POCKET GUIDE
FOR
Medical Assisting

Fourth Edition

Judy Kronenberger, RN, CMA, MEd
Associate Professor, Medical Assistant Technology
Sinclair Community College
Dayton, Ohio

Laura Southard Durham, BS, CMA
Medical Assisting Technologies Program Coordinator (Retired)
Forsyth Technical Community College
Winston-Salem, North Carolina

Denise Woodson, MA, MT(ASCP)SC
Academic Coordinator
Health Professions and Nursing
Smarthinking, Inc.
Richmond, Virginia

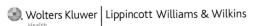
Wolters Kluwer | Lippincott Williams & Wilkins
Health
Philadelphia · Baltimore · New York · London
Buenos Aires · Hong Kong · Sydney · Tokyo

Acquisitions Editor: Kelley Squazzo
Product Manager: John Larkin
Marketing Manager: Shauna Kelley
Designer: Stephen Druding
Compositor: SPi Global

Fourth Edition

Copyright © 2012, 2009, 2005, 1999 Lippincott Williams and Wilkins

351 West Camden Street
Baltimore, MD 21201

Two Commerce Square
2001 Market Street
Philadelphia, PA 19103

Printed in China

Library of Congress Cataloging-in-Publication Data

Kronenberger, Judy.
  Lippincott Williams & Wilkins pocket guide for medical assisting / Judy Kronenberger, Laura Southard
  Durham, Denise Woodson.—4th ed.
     p. ; cm.
  Pocket guide for medical assisting
  Abridged version of: Lippincott Williams & Wilkins' comprehensive medical assisting / Judy Kronenberger.
  4th ed. c2011.
  Includes index.
  ISBN 978-1-4511-2037-0
  1. Durham, Laura Southard. II. Woodson, Denise. III. Kronenberger, Judy. Lippincott Williams & Wilkins'
  comprehensive medical assisting. IV. Title. V. Title: Pocket guide for medical assisting.
  [DNLM: 1. Physician Assistants—Handbooks. 2. Clinical Medicine—methods—Handbooks. 3. Medical
  Secretaries—Handbooks. 4. Practice Management, Medical—Handbooks. W 49]
  610.73'72069—dc23
                                                                                2011014497

To purchase additional copies of this book, call our customer service department at (800) 638-3030 or fax orders to (301) 223-2320. International customers should call (301) 223-2300.

Visit Lippincott Williams & Wilkins on the Internet: http://www.lww.com. Lippincott Williams & Wilkins customer service representatives are available from 8:30 am to 6:00 pm, EST.

9 8 7 6 5 4 3 2

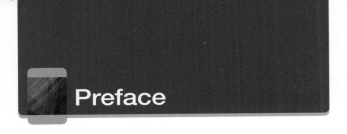

Preface

Lippincott Williams & Wilkins' Pocket Guide for Medical Assisting provides the essential information you need to make the transition from the classroom to the clinic as smooth and as stress-free as possible. The new streamlined, quick-reference format allows you to easily find key information to carry out clinical, administrative, and laboratory duties.

Lippincott Williams & Wilkins' Pocket Guide for Medical Assisting is organized into eight tabs:

1. Administrative Procedures
2. Clinical Procedures
3. Laboratory and Diagnostic Tests
4. Medication Administration
5. Surgical Procedures
6. Specialty Procedures
7. Emergency Procedures
8. Tools

Each tab is color-coded so you can clearly identify sections. Special features include "Warning" boxes, which describe situations that may pose an increased risk to you or your patient, and "Charting Examples" that present realistic samples of the information required for legal documentation.

Icons reminding you to follow Standard Precautions appear after the equipment list for each procedure and may include handwashing, gloving, personal protective equipment (PPE), or sharps and biohazard containers. Line drawings and photographs clarify key steps and visually enhance the procedures.

Vital reference material includes commonly prescribed medications, normal lab values, pain assessment tools, HIPAA resources, key English-to-Spanish health care phrases, a basic medical terminology refresher, commonly used abbreviations, Celsius-Fahrenheit conversions, metric equivalents, and more.

We hope you will use this compact, durable guide to perform with confidence in the administrative, clinical, and laboratory settings.

Judy Kronenberger
Laura Southard Durham
Denise Woodson

Icons Guide

 Handwashing

 Gloves

 Biohazardous

 PPE

 Sharps

Reviewers

Diana Alagna, RN
Medical Assistant Program Director
Medical Assisting Department
Branford Hall Career Institute
Southington, CT

Delena Austin, BTIS, CMA
Medical Assisting Program Coordinator
Health and Human Services Department
Macomb Community College
ClintonTownship, MI

Cheryl Charest
Medical Assistant, CET, Student Services
Coordinator
Medial Assistant Program
Premier Education Group
Manchester, NH

Anne Gailey, CMA (AAMA)
Medical Assisting Instructor
Medical Assisting Program
Ogeechee Technical College
Statesboro, GA

Marta Lopez, LM, CPM, RMA, BS
Program Coordinator/Faculty
Medical Assisting Department
Miami Dade College-Medical
Miami, FL

Paula Perkins, LPN, AABA, RMA
Manager, Vocational Programs
Stone Academy
Hamden, CT

Gregory Smith, MSW
Department Chair
Allied Health Department
Brown Mackie College - Tucson
Tucson, AZ

Stacey Wilson, BS, MHA
Program Chair
Medical Assistant Program
Cabarrus College of Health Sciences
Concord, NC

Contents

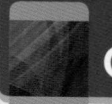

Specimen Collection and Microbiology

Immunology

Chemistry Testing

Administrative Procedures

Procedure 1-1 Incoming Telephone Calls

1. Answer within two rings.
2. Greet the caller and identify yourself and the medical office.
3. Determine the reason for the call and triage it.
4. Record the message, including:
   - Caller's name and telephone number
   - Date and time of call
   - Description of caller's concerns
   - Name of person to whom the message is routed
5. Tell the caller when to expect a return call.
6. Ask if the caller has any more questions or needs other help.
7. Allow the caller to disconnect first.
8. Put the message in an assigned place.

WARNING ⚠

Patients calling about medical emergencies (e.g., chest pain, short-ness of breath, loss of consciousness, profuse bleeding, etc.) should be directed to the nearest emergency room; follow protocol.

PATIENT APPOINTMENTS

Procedure 1-2 New Patient Appointments

1. Obtain the following information:
   - Patient's full name and correct spelling
   - Mailing address
   - Day and evening telephone numbers
   - Reason for the visit or chief complaint
   - Name of the referring physician
2. Explain the office's payment policy and ask the patient to bring insurance information.
3. Give directions to your office, if needed.
4. Ensure confidentiality by obtaining permission to call the patient at home or at work; chart this information.
5. Confirm the date and time of the appointment. *"Thank you for calling, Mr. Brown. We look forward to seeing you on Tuesday, December 10, at 2 P.M."*
6. Verify that you have placed the appointment on the right day and at the right time in the appointment system or book.
7. For referred patients: Obtain consent to request copies of pertinent medical records from the referring physician's office. Give these to your physician before the appointment.

Procedure 1-3 Established Patient Appointments

1. Determine the type of visit needed.
2. Review available appointments, then offer a specific time and date. *"Mrs. Chang, we can see you next Tuesday, the 15th, at 3:30 P.M. or Wednesday, the 16th, at 9:00 A.M."*
3. Place the patient's name and telephone number in the appointment schedule.
4. Restate the appointment day, date, and time.
5. If the patient is in the office, provide a completed appointment card.

Procedure 1-4 Referrals to an Outpatient Facility

Equipment
- Patient's chart
- Physician's order for services needed by the patient and reason for the services
- Patient's insurance card with referral information
- Referral form
- Directions to the referred provider's office

1. Handle any third-party payer requirements (e.g., precertification).
2. Have the patient choose a provider from the insurance company's preferred provider list.
3. Gather the following information before calling the referred provider:
   - Physician's name and telephone number
   - Patient's name, address, and telephone number
   - Reason for the call
   - Degree of urgency
   - Need for consultation or referral
4. Chart the date and time of the call and the name of the person you spoke with.
5. Ask to be notified if the patient misses the appointment (if this occurs, tell your physician and document this information in the patient's chart).
6. Give the patient the referred provider's name, address, and telephone number; the appointment date and time; and directions to the office.

Procedure 1-5 Admission to an Inpatient Facility

Equipment
- Patient's chart
- Physician's order with diagnosis
- Patient's insurance card
- Contact information for inpatient facility

1. Determine the inpatient facility where the admission will occur.
2. Gather the patient's demographic and insurance information.
3. Determine any precertification requirements.
4. Obtain the physician's diagnosis and the patient's exact needs for admission.
5. Call the inpatient facility's admissions department and give information from step 2.
6. Obtain instructions for the patient; provide this information in writing.
7. Give the patient the physician's orders for the hospital stay, for example, diet, medications, bed rest, etc.
8. Document time, place, etc., in patient's chart, including any precertification requirements completed.

MEDICAL RECORDS

Procedure 1-6 Creating a Medical File

Equipment
- File folder
- Metal fasteners
- Hole punch
- Five divider sheets with tabs
- Title, year, and alphabetic or numeric labels

1. Determine the file's name (e.g., patient's name, company name, or type of information to be stored).
2. Prepare a label with the file name *in unit order* (e.g., Lynn, Laila S., *not* Laila S. Lynn) and place it on the folder's tabbed edge.
3. Place a year label on the tab's top edge.
4. Place the appropriate alphabetic or numeric labels below the file name.

5. Apply any additional labels that your office uses (e.g., drug allergies, insurance, advance directives).
6. Punch holes and insert demographic and financial information on the left side of the chart using top fasteners.
7. Make tabs for H&P, Progress Notes, Medication Log, Correspondence, Test Results, etc.
8. Place pages behind appropriate tabs.

Procedure 1-7   Filing Medical Records

1. Check spelling of names on the chart and any single sheets to be placed in the folder.
2. Condition any single sheets.
3. Place sheets behind proper tabs.
4. Remove outguide.
5. Place the folder between the two appropriate existing folders.
6. Scan color coding to ensure that the charts in that section are in order.

BOX 1-1   Indexing Rules for Alphabetic Filing

* File by name according to last name, first name, and middle initial; treat each letter in the name as a separate unit. *Jamey L. Crowell should be filed as Crowell, Jamey L. and should come before Crowell, Jamie L.*
* Place professional initials after a full name. *John P. Bonnet, D.O., should be filed as Bonnet, John P., D.O.*
* Treat hyphenated names as one unit. *Bernadette M. Ryan-Nardone should be filed as Ryan-Nardone, Bernadette M. not as Nardone, Bernadette M. Ryan.*
* File abbreviated names as if they were spelled out. *Finnigan, Wm. should be filed as Finnigan, William, and St. James should be filed as Saint James.*

BOX 1-1 Indexing Rules for Alphabetic Filing (*Cont.*)

* File last names beginning with Mac and Mc in regular order or grouped together, per office preference.
* File a married woman's record by using her own first name. *Helen Johnston (Mrs. Kevin Johnston) should be filed as Johnston, Helen, not as Johnston, Kevin Mrs.*
* Use Jr. and Sr. when indexing and labeling the record.
* When names are identical, use the next unit, such as birth dates or the mother's maiden name. *Use Durham, Iran (2-4-94) and Durham, Iran (4-5-45).*
* Disregard apostrophes.
* Disregard articles (a, the), conjunctions (and, or), and prepositions (in, of) in filing.
* Treat letters in a company name as separate units. *For ASM, Inc., "A" is the first unit, "S" is the second unit, and "M" is the third unit.*

DOCUMENTATION

BOX 1-2 Documentation Guidelines

1. Ensure you have the correct patient chart. Double-check by asking for a birth date or social security number.
2. Document in ink.
3. Sign your complete name and credential.
4. Record the date of each entry.
5. Write legibly.
6. Check spelling, especially medical terms.
7. Use only accepted abbreviations.
8. Use quotation marks to signify the patient's own words. *Example: "My head is killing me."*
9. Document as soon as possible after completing a task.

BOX 1-2 Documentation Guidelines (*Cont.*)

10. Document missed appointments.
11. Document calls for appointment reminders.
12. Document any telephone conversations with the patient.
13. Be honest. If you have given a wrong medication or performed the wrong procedure, document it immediately after notifying the appropriate supervisor, then complete an incident report (see below).
14. Electronic charting: You can click on an icon to make a correction in the electronic chart, but the original information is not deleted. For example, if you discover that you have entered the wrong date of birth after the patient's information has been saved, you can correct it, but most systems allow only certain users to make changes in the saved database.

WARNING

- Never diagnose a condition. *Do not write* "Patient has pharyngitis." Instead write "Patient c/o a sore throat."
- Never document for someone else, and never ask someone else to document for you.
- Never document false information.
- Never delete, erase, scribble over, or white-out information in the medical record. If you do make an error, draw a single line through it, initial it, and date it. Then write the word "correction" and document the correct information.

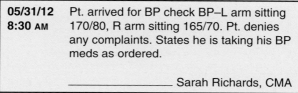

| 05/31/12 8:30 AM | Pt. arrived for BP check BP–L arm sitting 170/80, R arm sitting 165/70. Pt. denies any complaints. States he is taking his BP meds as ordered. |
| | _____ Sarah Richards, CMA |

Figure 1-1. Narrative charting example.

Correct

9-15-12	Pt. Called to cancel appt. for recheck of UTI on 9-16-08. States she is feeling better. Advised to keep appointment, since Dr. Smith wants to repeat a urinalysis to see if her bladder infection has cleared up. Pt. states, "I don't see any sense in that; I'm not coming". Advised Dr. Smith. Fred Lane, CMA

Incorrect

9-15-12	Pt. called to cancel appt. Fred Lane, CMA

Figure 1-2. Right and wrong chart entries.

When correcting a charting error, draw a single line through the error, initial it, date it, and document the correct information.

left 05/15/12 TW
05/15/12 Patient presents today complaining of pain in ~~right~~ eye. Tracy Wiles, CMA

Figure 1-3. Correcting an error in the medical record.

Procedure 1-8 Bank Deposits

Equipment
- Calculator with tape
- Currency, coins, checks
- Deposit slip
- Endorsement stamp
- Deposit envelope or bank bag

1. Separate cash from checks.
2. Arrange bills face up and sorted, largest denomination on top.
3. Record the total in the cash block on the deposit slip.
4. Endorse each check with "For Deposit Only" stamp.
5. Record the amount of each check beside an identifying number on the deposit slip.
6. Total and record the amount of all checks.
7. Subtotal and record the amount of all cash and checks.
8. Record the total amount of the deposit on the checkbook register.
9. Copy both sides of the deposit slip for office records.
10. Place the cash, checks, and completed deposit slip in an envelope or bank bag for transporting to the bank.

Procedure 1-9 Reconcile a Bank Statement

Equipment
- Bank statement
- Reconciliation worksheet
- Calculator
- Pen

1. Compare the new statement's opening balance with the previous statement's closing balance.
2. List the bank balance on the reconciliation worksheet.
3. Compare the check entries on the statement with the entries in the check register. Place a check mark beside each check listed as paid on the statement.
4. List the amounts of outstanding checks; total.
5. Subtract from the checkbook balance items that appear on the statement but not in the checkbook (e.g., automatic payments, service charges, withdrawals).
6. Add to the balance any deposits not shown on the bank statement.
7. Ensure that the balances in the checkbook and the bank statement agree.

Procedure 1-10 Maintain a Petty Cash Account

1. Count the money in the petty cash box.
2. Total the amounts of all vouchers to determine expenditures.

3. Subtract the amount of receipts from the original amount in petty cash. (This should equal the amount of cash remaining in the box.)
4. After balancing the cash against the receipts, write a check for the amount of cash that was used.
5. Sort and record all vouchers to the appropriate accounts.
6. File the list of vouchers and receipts attached.
7. Place cash in petty cash box.

Procedure 1-11 Check Writing

On the check register, fill out:
- Check number
- Date
- Payee
- Amount
- Previous balance
- New balance

On the check, fill out:
- Date
- Payee
- Amount (using numerals)
- Amount (written out; record cents as a fraction with 100 as the denominator)
- Obtain required signature(s).

WRITTEN COMMUNICATION

Benjamin Matthews, M.D.
999 Oak Road, Suite 313
Middletown, Connecticut 06457   ①
860-344-6000

February 2, 2012   ②

Dr. Adam Meza
Medical Director   ③
Family Practice Associates
134 N. Tater Drive
West Hartford, Connecticut 06157

Re: Ms. Beatrice Staley   ④

Dear Dr.Meza: ⑤

Thank you for asking me to evaluate Ms. Staley. I agree with your diagnosis of rheumatoid arthritis.
Her prodromal symptoms include vague articular pain and stiffness, weight loss and general malaise.
Ms. Staley states that the joint discomfort is most prominent in the mornings, gradually improving
thrugihout the day.

My physical examination shows a 40-year-old female patient in good health. Heart sounds normal,
no murmurs or gallops noted. Lung sounds clear. Enlarged lymph nodes were noted. Abdomen
soft, bowel sounds present, and the spleen was not enlarged. Extremities showed subcutaneous
nodules and flexion contractures on both hands.

⑥

Laboratory findings were indicative of rheumatoid arthritis. See attached laboratory data. I do
not feel x-rays are warranted at this time.

My recommendations are to continue Ms. Staley on salicylate therapy, rest and physical therapy.
I suggest that you have Ms. Staley attend physical therapy at the American Rehabilitation Center
on Main Street.

Thank you for this interesting consultation.

Yours truly,   ⑦

Benjamin Matthews, MD   ⑧
Benjamin Matthews, MD

BM/es   ⑨

Enc. (2)   ⑩

c: Dr. Samuel Adams   ⑪

Figure 1-4. Business letter components. This letter is done in full block
format and contains these elements: (1) letterhead, (2) date, (3) inside
address, (4) subject line, (5) salutation, (6) body, (7) closing, (8) signature
and typed name, (9) identification line, (10) enclosure, (11) copy.

BOX 1-3   Basic Punctuation and Grammar

Punctuation
- Period (.)—Used at the end of sentences and after abbreviations.
- Comma (,)—Separates words or phrases that are part of a series of three or more.
- Semicolon (;)—Separates a long list of items in a series and independent clauses not joined by a conjunction.
- Colon (:)—Used to introduce a series of items, to follow formal salutations, and to separate the hours from minutes indicating time.
- Apostrophe (')—Denotes omissions of letters and the possessive case of nouns.
- Quotation marks (" ")—Set off spoken dialogue, some titles (e.g., journal articles), and words used in a special way.
- Parentheses [( )]—Indicate a part of a sentence that is not part of the main sentence but is essential for the meaning of the sentence. Also used to enclose a number, for confirmation, that is spelled out in a sentence.
- Ellipsis (. . .)—Used in place of a period to indicate a prolonged continuation of a conversation or list.
- Diagonal (/)—Used in abbreviations (c/o), dates (2012/2013), fractions (3/4), and to indicate two or more options (AM/FM).

Sentence Structure
- Avoid run-on sentences.
- Ensure that the verb always agrees with its subject in number and person.
- Use correct pronouns.
- Use adjectives only when they add an important message.

Capitalization
- Capitalize the first word in a sentence, proper nouns, the pronoun "I," book titles, and known geographical names.
- Capitalize names of persons, holidays, and trademarked items.
- Do not capitalize expressions of time (A.M. and P.M.).

BOX 1-4 Rules for Pluralizing Medical Terms

A add an E
UM changes to A
US changes to I
ON changes to A
IS changes to ES or IDES

AX or IX change the X to C
  and add ES
EX changes to ICES
EN drop the EN and add INA
MA changes to MATA
NX or YNX change to NGES

bulla becomes bullae
ovum becomes ova
bronchus becomes bronchi
phenomenon becomes phenomena
testis becomes testes, epididymis
  becomes epididymides
thorax becomes thoraces

index becomes indices
lumen becomes lumina
carcinoma becomes carcinomata
phalanx becomes phalanges, larynx
  becomes larynges

INCIDENT REPORTS

BOX 1-5 When to Complete an Incident Report

The following situations require an incident report:
* All medication errors
* All patient, visitor, and employee falls
* Drawing blood from the wrong patient
* Mislabeled blood tubes or specimens
* Incorrect surgical instrument counts following surgery
* Employee needlesticks
* Workers'compensation injuries

BOX 1-6 **What to Include on an Incident Report**

- Injured party's name, address, and phone number
- Injured party's birth date and sex
- Date, time, and location of the incident
- Brief description of the incident and what was done to correct it
- Any diagnostic procedures or treatments that were needed
- Patient examination findings, if applicable
- Witnesses' names and addresses, if applicable
- Signature and title of person completing form
- Physician's and supervisor's signatures as per policy

BOX 1-7 **Guidelines for Completing an Incident Report**

1. State only the facts. Do not draw conclusions or place blame.
2. Write legibly and sign your name clearly, including your title.
3. Complete the form within 24 hours of the event.
4. Do not leave any blank spaces on the form. If a section of the report does not apply, write n/a (not applicable).

WARNING

- Never photocopy an incident report for your own personal record.
- Never place the incident report in the patient's chart.
- Never document in the patient's chart that an incident report was completed, only document the event.

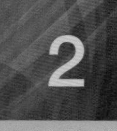

Clinical Procedures

2

Procedure 2-1 Medical Aseptic Handwashing

Equipment
- Liquid soap
- Paper towels
- Orangewood manicure stick
- Waste can

1. Remove rings and wristwatch, or push wristwatch up onto your forearm.
2. Stand close to the sink without touching it.
3. Wet your hands and wrists under warm running water and apply liquid soap.
4. Lather, then rub the soap between your fingers.
5. Scrub the palm of one hand with the fingertips of the other hand, then reverse; scrub each wrist.
6. Rinse thoroughly, holding hands lower than elbows; avoid touching the inside of the sink.
7. Clean under fingernails with orangewood stick.
8. Reapply soap and rewash hands and wrists.
9. Rinse thoroughly again while holding hands lower than wrists and elbows.
10. Dry hands gently with a paper towel; discard the towel and orangewood stick.
11. Use a dry paper towel to turn off the faucets; discard.

TABLE 2-1 Comparing Medical and Surgical Asepsis		
	Medical Asepsis	Surgical Asepsis
Definition	Destroys microorganisms after they leave the body	Destroys microorganisms before they enter the body
Purpose	Prevents transmission of microorganisms from one person to another	Maintains sterility when entering a normally sterile part of the body
When used	Used when coming in contact with a body part that is not normally sterile	Used when entering a normally sterile part of the body
Differences in handwashing technique	Hands and wrists are washed for 1 to 2 minutes; no brush is used. Hands are held down to rinse so that water runs off fingertips. A paper towel is used for drying.	Hands and forearms are washed for 5 to 10 minutes; a brush is used for hands, arms, and nails. Hands are held up to rinse so that water runs off elbows. A sterile towel is used for drying.

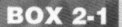 **Maintaining Medical Asepsis**

- Avoid touching your clothing with soiled linen, table paper, supplies, or instruments. Roll used table paper or linens inward with the clean surface outward.
- Clean tables, counters, and other surfaces frequently, and immediately after contamination.
- Always consider the floor to be contaminated. Discard any item dropped onto the floor or clean it to its former level of asepsis before using it.
- Always consider blood and body fluids to be contaminated. Follow OSHA and CDC guidelines to prevent disease transmission.

 Standard Precautions: Do's and Don'ts

DO:
- Wash your hands with soap and water after touching blood, body fluids, secretions, and other contaminated items, even if gloves were worn.
- Use an alcohol-based hand rub (foam, lotion, or gel) to decontaminate hands if they are not visibly dirty or contaminated.
- Wear clean, nonsterile examination gloves when anticipating contact with blood, body fluids, secretions, mucous membranes, damaged skin, and contaminated items.
- Change gloves between procedures on the same patient after exposure to potentially infective material.
- Wear equipment to protect your eyes, nose, and mouth, and wear a disposable gown or apron to prevent soiling your clothes when performing procedures that may splash or spray blood, body fluids, or secretions.
- Take precautions to avoid injuries before, during, and after procedures in which needles, scalpels, or other sharp instruments have been used on a patient.

Procedure 2-2 Removing Contaminated Gloves

1. Grasp the glove of your nondominant hand at the palm and pull it away (Fig. 2-1).
2. Slide your hand out while rolling the glove into the palm of your gloved hand (Figs. 2-2 and 2-3).
3. Holding the soiled glove in your gloved hand, slip your ungloved fingers under the cuff of the gloved hand. Do not touch the outside of the glove (Fig. 2-4).
4. Stretch the glove up and away from your hand; turn it inside out as you pull it off with the other glove balled up inside (Fig. 2-5).
5. Discard into a biohazard waste container.
6. Wash your hands.

19

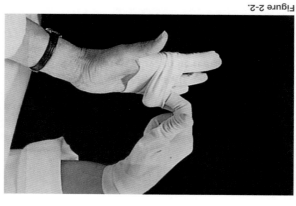

Figure 2-1.

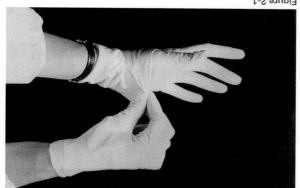

Figure 2-2.

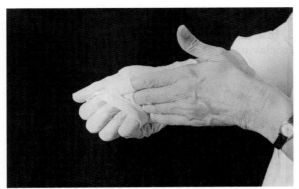

Figure 2-3.

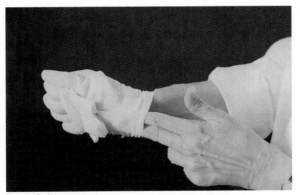

Figure 2-4.

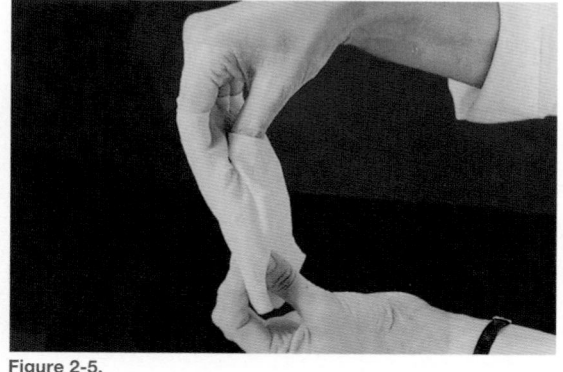

Figure 2-5.

Procedure 2-3 Cleaning Biohazardous Spills

Equipment
- Commercially prepared germicide *or* 1:10 bleach solution
- Paper towels
- Chemical absorbent
- Disposable shoe coverings

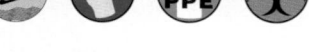

1. Put on gloves, PPE, and protective shoe coverings.
2. Apply chemical absorbent to spill and clean it up with paper towels; avoid splashing.
3. Discard paper towels and absorbent material in a biohazard bag.

4. Spray the area with commercial germicide or bleach solution and wipe with paper towels. Discard towels in a biohazard bag.
5. With your gloves on, remove PPE and shoe coverings; discard in biohazard bag or handle per office policy.
6. Place the biohazard bag in an appropriate waste receptacle.
7. Discard gloves and wash your hands.

BOX 2-3 **Disposing of Infectious Waste**

- Use regular waste containers only for nonbiohazardous waste, for example, paper, plastic, disposable tray wrappers, packaging material, unused gauze, and exam table paper.
- Use separate containers for different types of biohazardous waste, for example, don't put bandages in sharps containers.
- Use only approved biohazard containers.
- Fill sharps containers two-thirds full before disposing of them.
- Before moving filled biohazard containers, secure the bag or top with the appropriate closure.
- If the container's outer surface is contaminated, put on clean exam gloves, secure the container within another approved container, and wash your hands when done.
- *Never* discard sharps in plastic bags; these are not puncture resistant and injury may occur.

Procedure 2-4 Sanitizing Equipment for Disinfection or Sterilization

Equipment
- Instruments or equipment to be sanitized
- Soap and water
- Small handheld scrub brush

23

1. Put on gloves, gown, and eye protection.
2. Take apart any removable sections.
3. Check that items operate properly.
4. Rinse instruments with cool water.
5. Force streams of soapy water through tubular or grooved instruments.
6. Use a hot, soapy solution to dissolve fats or lubricants.
7. After soaking for 5 to 10 minutes, use friction with a soft brush or gauze to wipe down the instrument and loosen microorganisms. Do not use abrasive materials on delicate instruments and equipment.
8. Open and close the jaws of scissors or forceps to ensure that all material has been removed.
9. Rinse and dry well before autoclaving or soaking in disinfectant.
10. Disinfect or discard brushes, gauze, and solution.

Procedure 2-5 Wrapping Instruments for Sterilization in an Autoclave

Equipment
- Instruments or equipment to be sterilized
- Wrapping material
- Autoclave tape
- Sterilization indicator
- Black or blue ink pen

1. Check that items to be sterilized operate properly.
2. Select appropriate wrapping material.
3. On the autoclave tape, write the package contents or the name of the instrument to be wrapped, the date, and your initials.
4. When using autoclave wrapping material made of cotton muslin or special paper:
   - Lay the material diagonally on a flat, clean, dry surface.
   - Center the instrument on the wrapping material with the ratchets or handles open.
   - Include a sterilization indicator (Fig. 2-6).

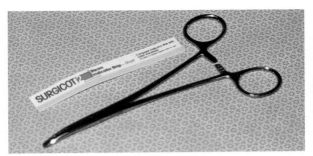

Figure 2-6.

5. Fold the first flap at the bottom of the diagonal wrap up, and fold back the corner making a tab (Fig. 2-7).
6. Fold the left corner of the wrap, then the right, each making a tab for opening the package. Secure the package with autoclave tape (Fig. 2-8).
7. Fold the top corner down, tucking the tab under the material (Fig. 2-9).
8. Secure with autoclave tape.

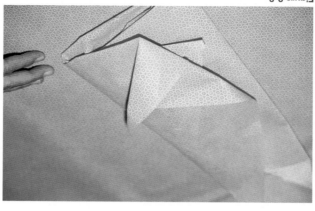

Figure 2-7.

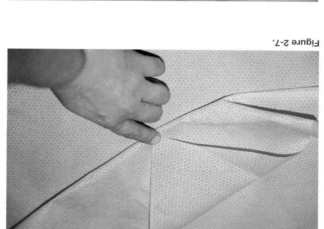

Figure 2-8.

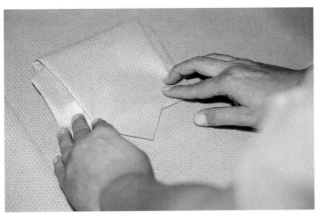

Figure 2-9.

Procedure 2-6 Operating an Autoclave

Equipment
- Sanitized and wrapped instruments or equipment
- Distilled water
- Autoclave operating manual

1. Assemble the equipment, the wrapped articles, and the sterilization indicator in each package.
2. Check the autoclave reservoir level; add more distilled water if needed.
3. Add water to the autoclave's internal chamber to the fill line.
4. Load the autoclave:
   - Place trays and packs on their sides 1 to 3 inches apart.
   - Put containers on their side with the lid off.
   - In mixed loads, place hard objects on the bottom shelf and softer packs on the top racks.

5. Follow the machine's operating instructions (most use this protocol):
   • Close the door and secure or lock it.
   • Turn the machine on.
   • Set the timer when the temperature gauge reaches the required point (usually 250°F).
   • Vent the chamber when the cycle is over.
   • Release the pressure to a safe level.
   • Crack the door to allow additional drying.
6. Remove items when the load has cooled.
7. Check the separately wrapped sterilization indicator, if used, for proper sterilization.
8. Store the items in a clean, dry, dust-free area for 30 days.
9. Clean the autoclave per manufacturer's suggestions.

WARNING ⚠

If the indicator does not show proper sterilization, consider the items *not* sterile and reprocess the load.

PATIENT CARE

Procedure 2-7   Obtaining a Medical History

Equipment
   • Medical history form
   • Pen

1. Review the medical history form.
2. Take the patient to a private and comfortable room.
3. Sit across from the patient and maintain frequent eye contact.
4. Introduce yourself and explain the interview's purpose.
5. Interview the patient, documenting all responses.
6. Determine the CC and PI.
7. Listen actively and avoid making judgments.

8. Explain any examinations or procedures scheduled for the visit.
9. Thank the patient and offer to answer questions.

Procedure 2-8 Measuring Weight

Equipment
- Calibrated balance beam scale, digital scale, or dial scale
- Paper towel
- Patient's chart

1. Ensure the scale is properly balanced at zero.
2. Escort the patient to the scale and place a paper towel on it.
3. Have the patient remove shoes, heavy outerwear, and put down purse.
4. Have the patient face forward on the scale, standing on the paper towel, not touching or holding onto anything.
5. Weigh the patient:
   - *Balance beam scale:* Slide counterweights on bottom and top bars from zero to approximate weight. To obtain measurement, balance bar must hang freely at exact midpoint. Return the bars to zero.
   - *Digital scale:* Read weight displayed on digital screen.
   - *Dial scale:* Indicator arrow rests at patient's weight.
6. Assist the patient from the scale if necessary; watch for balance difficulties.
7. Discard the paper towel.
8. Record the weight.

BOX 2-4 **Converting Between Pounds and Kilograms**

Note: 1 kg = 2.2 lb
* To change pounds to kilograms: Divide the number of pounds by 2.2
* To change kilograms to pounds: Multiply the number of kilograms by 2.2

Procedure 2-9 Measuring Height

Equipment
* Scale with a ruler
* Patient's chart

1. Have the patient remove shoes and stand straight and erect on the scale, back to the ruler, heels together, eyes straight ahead.
2. Lower the measuring bar until it touches the patient's head.
3. Read the measurement.
4. Assist the patient from the scale if necessary; watch for balance difficulties.
5. Record the height.

BOX 2-5 **Converting Between Inches and Centimeters**

Note: 1 inch = 2.5 cm
* To convert inches to centimeters: Multiply the number of inches by 2.5
* To convert centimeters to inches: Divide the number of centimeters by 2.5

Procedure 2-10   Assisting with the Adult Physical Exam

Equipment
- Stethoscope
- Ophthalmoscope
- Otoscope
- Penlight
- Tuning fork
- Nasal speculum
- Tongue blade
- Percussion hammer
- Water-soluble lubricant
- Examination light
- Patient gown and draping supplies
- Patient's chart

1. Prepare the examination room and equipment.
2. Obtain and record the medical history and chief complaint.
3. Record vital signs, height, weight, and visual acuity.
4. If required, instruct the patient to obtain a urine specimen.
5. Instruct the patient to disrobe and put the gown on.
6. Help the patient sit on the table edge; drape the lap and legs.
7. Place the chart outside the examination room and notify the physician.
8. Hand the physician the instruments as needed and position the patient appropriately (Fig. 2-10).
   (a) Begin with instruments needed to examine the following:
   - Head and neck   Stethoscope
   - Eyes   Ophthalmoscope, penlight
   - Ears   Otoscope, tuning fork
   - Nose   Penlight, nasal speculum
   - Sinuses   Penlight

| • Mouth | Tongue blade, penlight |
| • Throat | Glove, tongue blade, laryngeal mirror, penlight |

(b) Help the patient drop the gown to the waist for chest and upper back examination. Hand the physician the stethoscope.

(c) Help the patient pull the gown up and remove the drape from the legs for reflex testing. Hand the physician the percussion hammer.

(d) Help the patient lie supine, opening the gown at the top to expose the chest again. Drape the waist, abdomen, and legs. Hand the physician the stethoscope.

(e) Cover the patient's chest and lower the drape to expose the abdomen. Hand the physician the stethoscope.

(f) Assist with the genital and rectal examinations. Hand the patient tissues following these examinations.

For female patients:

- Assist to the lithotomy position and drape appropriately.
- For examination of the genitalia and internal reproductive organs: provide a glove, lubricant, speculum, microscope slides or liquid prep solution, and Ayres spatula or brush.
- For the rectal examination: provide a glove, lubricant, and fecal occult blood test slide.

For male patients:

- Help the patient stand and have him bend over the examination table.
- For a hernia examination: provide a glove.
- For a rectal examination: provide a glove, lubricant, and fecal occult blood test slide
- For a prostate examination: provide a glove and lubricant

(g) With the patient standing, the physician can assess the legs, gait, coordination, and balance.

9. Help the patient sit at the table edge.

10. Perform any follow-up procedures or treatments.

11. Allow the patient to dress in private.
12. Answer any questions, reinforce physician instructions, and provide patient education.
13. Escort the patient to the front desk.
14. Clean or dispose of used equipment and supplies.
15. Prepare the room for the next patient.
16. Wash your hands and record any physician instructions.
17. Note any specimens and indicate test results or the laboratory where the specimens are being sent.

Figure 2-10. Patient exam positions. **(A)** The erect or standing position. The patient stands erect facing forward with the arms at the sides. **(B)** The sitting position. The patient sits erect at the end of the examination table with the feet supported on a footrest or stool. **(C)** The supine position. The patient lies on the back with arms at the sides. A pillow may be placed under the head for comfort. **(D)** The dorsal recumbent position. The patient is supine with the legs separated, knees bent, and feet flat on the table. **(E)** The lithotomy position, similar to the dorsal recumbent position but with the patient's feet in stirrups rather than flat on the table. The stirrups should be level with each other and about 1 foot out from the edge of the table. The patient's feet are moved into or out of the stirrups at the same time to prevent back strain. **(F)** The Sims position. The patient lies on the left side with the left arm and shoulder behind the body, right leg and arm sharply flexed on the table, and left knee slightly flexed. **(G)** The prone position. The patient lies on the abdomen with the head supported and turned to one side. The arms may be under the head or by the sides, whichever is more comfortable. **(H)** Knee-chest position. The patient kneels on the table with the arms and chest on the table, hips in the air, and back straight. (I) Fowler's position. The patient is half-sitting with the head of the examination table elevated 80 to 90 degrees. **(J)** Semi-Fowler position. The patient is in a half-sitting position with the head of the table elevated 30 to 45 degrees and the knees slightly bent. **(K)** Trendelenburg position. The patient lies on the back with arms straight at either side and the head of the bed is lowered with the head lower than the hips; the legs are elevated at approximately 45 degrees.

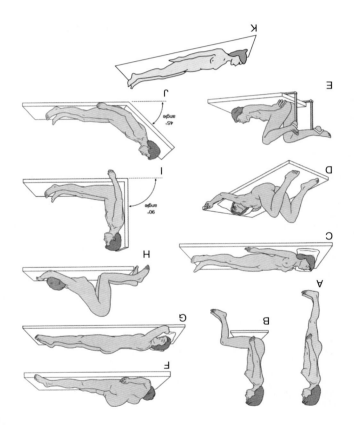

Procedure 2-11 Using an Electronic Thermometer

Equipment
- Electronic thermometer with oral or rectal probe
- Disposable probe covers
- Patient's chart

1. Choose the most appropriate method (oral, axillary, or rectal).
2. Attach the appropriate probe to the unit.
3. Insert the probe into a cover.
4. Position the thermometer appropriately. (For rectal temperature: wear gloves, apply lubricant to probe cover, and hold the probe in place.)
5. Remove the probe after the thermometer "beeps."
6. Note the reading.
7. Discard the probe cover.
8. Replace the probe into the unit.
9. Remove gloves (if any), wash your hands, and record the procedure.
10. Return the unit and probe to the charging base.

WARNING❗
- Avoid taking oral temperatures for patients who are postoperative for oral surgery, have seizure disorders, are receiving oxygen, are mouth breathers, or are congested.
- Avoid taking rectal temperatures for patients who are postoperative for rectal surgery, have seizure or cardiac disorders, or for children under age 2.

Procedure 2-12 Using a Tympanic Thermometer

Equipment
- Tympanic thermometer
- Disposable probe covers
- Patient's chart

1. Insert the ear probe into a cover.
2. Place the end of the probe into the patient's ear canal.
   For adults: Straighten the ear canal by pulling the outer ear
      up and back.
   For children under age 3: Pull the outer ear down and back.
3. Press the button on the thermometer and wait for the
   reading to display.
4. Remove the probe and note the reading.
5. Discard the probe cover.
6. Wash your hands and record the procedure.
7. Return the unit to the charging base.

TABLE **2-2**	Temperature Comparisons	
	Fahrenheit	Centigrade
Oral	98.6°	37.0°
Rectal	99.6° (R)	37.6°
Axillary	97.6° (A)	36.4°
Tympanic	98.6° (T)	37.0°

Procedure 2-13 Using a Temporal Artery Thermometer

Equipment
- Temporal artery thermometer
- Alcohol wipe
- Patient's chart

1. Make sure the patient's skin is dry.
2. Place the probe end of the handheld unit on the patient's forehead.
3. Depress the on/off button, move the thermometer across and down the forehead, and release the on/off button with the unit over the temporal artery.
4. Note the reading on the digital display screen.
5. Disinfect the end of the thermometer.
6. Wash your hands and record the procedure.
7. Return the unit to the charging base.

PULSE

Procedure 2-14 Measuring Radial Pulse

Equipment
- Watch with a sweeping second hand
- Patient's chart

2
Clinical

1. Position the patient with the arm relaxed and supported.
2. With the index, middle, and ring fingers of your dominant hand, press firmly with your fingertips to feel the pulse; do not obliterate it.
3. Measure the pulse.
   - Regular pulse: Count it for 30 seconds. Multiply the number of pulsations by 2 since the pulse is always recorded as beats per minute.
   - Irregular pulse: Count it for a full 60 seconds.
4. Record the rate. Also chart irregular rhythm or thready or bounding volume.

TABLE 2-3	Variations in Pulse Rate by Age
Age	Beats per Minute
Birth to 1 year	110–170
1–10 years	90–110
10–16 years	80–95
16 years to midlife	70–80
Elderly adult	55–70

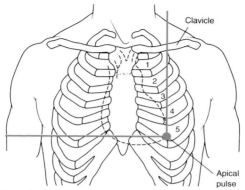

Figure 2-11. Finding the apical pulse site.

Clavicle

Apical pulse

Procedure 2-15 Assessing the Pulse Using a Doppler Unit

Equipment
- Doppler unit
- Coupling agent or transmission gel
- Watch with sweep second hand

1. Apply coupling agent or transmission gel to the probe.
2. Turn the machine on.
3. Hold the probe at a 45-degree angle. Avoid obliterating the pulse (Fig. 2-12).
4. Position the probe so the artery sound is dominant.
5. Assess the rate, rhythm, and volume.
6. Record the measurement.
7. Clean the patient's skin and probe with warm water.

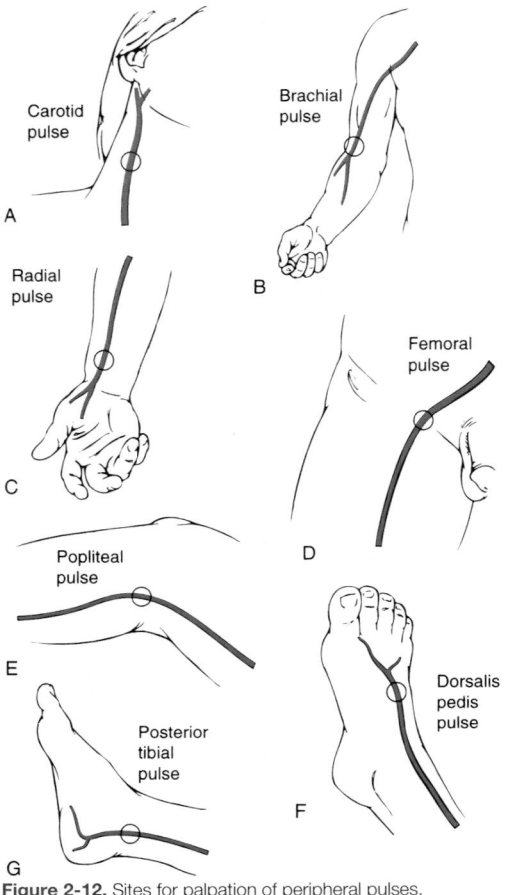

Figure 2-12. Sites for palpation of peripheral pulses.

Procedure 2-16 Measuring Respirations

Equipment
- Watch with a sweeping second hand
- Patient's chart

Note: Measure respirations immediately after counting the radial pulse.

1. Count a complete rise and fall of the chest as one respiration. (Some patients have abdominal movement rather than chest movement during respirations.)
2. Count respirations.
   - Regular breathing pattern: Count the respiratory rate for 30 seconds and multiply by 2.
   - Irregular breathing pattern: Count for a full 60 seconds.
3. Record the rate. Also chart irregular rhythm and note any unusual or abnormal sounds.

TABLE **2-4**	Variations in Respiration Ranges by Age
Age	Respirations per Minute
Infant	20+
Child	18–20
Adult	12–20

TABLE **2-5**	Abnormal Respiratory Patterns
Pattern	Description
Apnea	No respirations
Bradypnea	Slow respirations
Cheyne-Stokes	Rhythmic cycles of dyspnea or hyperpnea subsiding gradually into periods of apnea
Dyspnea	Difficult or labored respirations
Hypopnea	Shallow respirations
Hyperpnea	Deep respirations
Kussmaul	Fast and deep respirations
Orthopnea	Inability to breathe in other than a sitting or standing position
Tachypnea	Fast respirations

BLOOD PRESSURE

Procedure 2-17   Measuring Blood Pressure

Equipment
- Sphygmomanometer
- Stethoscope
- Patient's chart

1. Position the patient with the arm supported, at heart level.
2. Expose the arm.
3. Palpate the brachial pulse.
4. Center the cuff over the brachial artery.
5. Wrap the cuff around the arm and secure it.
6. With the air pump in your dominant hand and the valve between your thumb and forefinger, tighten the screw.
7. While palpating the brachial pulse, inflate the cuff. Note the point or number on the dial or mercury column at which brachial pulse is no longer felt.
8. Deflate the cuff. Wait at least 30 seconds before reinflating.
9. Hold the stethoscope diaphragm firmly against the brachial artery while taking the blood pressure and listening carefully.
10. Turn the screw to close the valve; inflate the cuff. Pump the valve bulb to about 30 mm Hg above the number felt during step 7.
11. With the cuff properly inflated, turn the valve counter-clockwise to release air at about 2 to 4 mm Hg per second.
12. Note the point on the gauge at which you hear the first clear tapping sound (systolic sound, or Korotkoff I).
13. Continue to listen and deflate the cuff.
14. When you hear the last sound, note the reading and quickly deflate the cuff.
15. Remove the cuff and press the air from the bladder.
16. Put the equipment away and wash your hands.
17. Record the reading. Note systolic over diastolic, which arm was used (120/80 LA), and position (if other than sitting).

WARNING ⚠️
- Never immediately reinflate the blood pressure cuff; always wait 1 to 2 minutes.
- Never attempt to assess BP in a patient's arm used for a dialysis shunt.
- Avoid limbs with edema, a heparin lock, or injuries; avoid the affected arm after a mastectomy.
- Notify the physician immediately if the pressure reads above 140/90 or below 100/50.

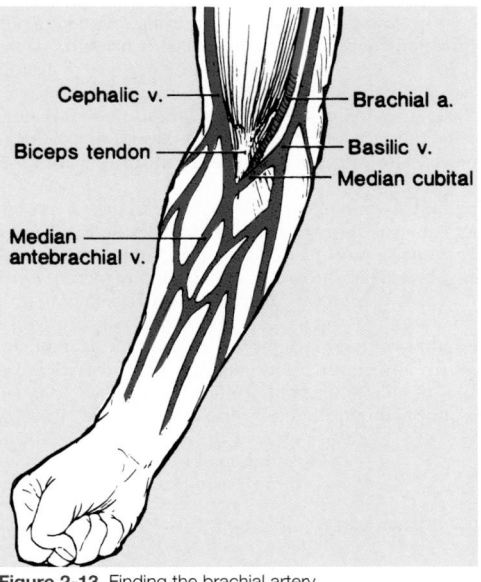

Figure 2-13. Finding the brachial artery.

TABLE 2-6	Blood Pressure Ranges		
	Systolic BP		Diastolic BP
Normal	<120 mm Hg	and	<80 mm Hg
Prehypertension	120–139 mm Hg	or	80–89 mm Hg
Hypertension, Stage I	140–159 mm Hg	or	90–99 mm Hg
Hypertension Stage II	≥160 mm Hg	or	≥100 mg Hg

From U.S. Department of Health and Human Services, National Institutes of
Health, National Heart, Lung, and Blood Institute.

TABLE 2-7	Five Phases of Blood Pressure
Phase	Sounds
I	Faint tapping heard as the cuff deflates (systolic blood pressure)
II	Soft swishing
III	Rhythmic, sharp, distinct tapping
IV	Soft tapping that becomes faint
V	Last sound (diastolic blood pressure)

BOX 2-6 Causes of Errors in Blood Pressure Readings

- Wrapping the cuff improperly
- Failing to keep the patient's arm at heart level
- Failing to support the patient's arm on a stable surface
- Recording auscultatory gap for diastolic pressure
- Failing to maintain the gauge at eye level
- Pulling the patient's sleeve up tightly above the cuff
- Listening through clothing
- Allowing the cuff to deflate too rapidly or too slowly
- Failing to wait 1 to 2 minutes before rechecking

CHARTING EXAMPLE

| 08/21/08 10:00 AM | T 99.6 (O) P 88 R 24 BP 136/86 (R) arm, sitting Ht. 5'7" Wt. 165# CC: c/o sore throat ×2 days. Denies fever, chills. Also c/o nasalcongestion with clear drainage ×1 week. |

——————————— S. Medina, RMA

Laboratory and Diagnostic Tests

Procedure 3-1 Venipuncture

Equipment
- Multisample needle and adaptor or winged infusion set
- Evacuated tubes
- Tourniquet
- Sterile gauze pads
- Bandages
- 70% alcohol pad
- Permanent marker or pen

1. Double-check the requisition slip.
2. Assemble equipment and check the tubes' expiration dates.
3. For fasting specimens, ask when the patient last ate or drank anything besides water.
4. Put on gloves or other PPE.
5. For *evacuated tube collection:* Break the needle cover seal. Thread the sleeved needle into the adaptor.
6. For winged infusion set collection: Extend the tubing. Thread the sleeved needle into the adaptor.
7. *For both methods:* Tap the tubes to dislodge the additive. Insert the tube into the adaptor.
8. Have the patient sit with arm supported.
9. Apply the tourniquet 3 to 4 inches above the elbow. Secure it with half-bow knot, tails extending upward.

47

10. Have the patient make a fist and hold it.
11. Palpate vein, then release tourniquet. Have the patient release fist.
12. Cleanse the site; let dry or dry it with sterile gauze.
13. Reapply tourniquet and have the patient make a fist.
14. Remove the needle cover.
15. Anchor the vein.
16. Insert the needle at 15- to 30-degree angle. (Use lesser angle for winged infusion set collections.)
17. Push the tube onto the needle inside the adaptor.
18. Allow the tube to fill to capacity.
19. Release the tourniquet and have the patient release fist.
20. When blood flow stops, remove tube from the adaptor and insert the next tube if needed.
21. Remove tube from the adaptor.
22. Withdraw needle and place a sterile gauze pad over the puncture site.
23. Activate the safety device and apply pressure to the site.
24. Gently invert tubes containing anticoagulants. Do not shake.
25. Label the tubes.
26. Apply dressing and bandage.
27. Release the patient when bleeding has stopped.
28. Care for or discard equipment and clean the work area.
29. Remove PPE and wash your hands.
30. Test, transfer, or store the blood specimen according to office policy.
31. Record the procedure.

CHARTING EXAMPLE

05/31/08	OP venipuncture for platelet count,
10:00 AM	dx code ###.## per Dr. Jacobs.
	———————————— J. Simpson, RMA

WARNING ⚠️
- Do not puncture the top of the vacuum tube before inserting the needle into the patient. Doing this removes the vacuum, so the specimen will not flow into the tube even if the venipuncture is accurate.
- If you accidentally enter an artery, keep pressure on the site for at least 5 minutes. Note it on the patient's chart.

BOX 3-1 **Order of Draw**

Tube Stopper Color
Yellow
Red
Light blue
Red and gray rubber
Gold plastic
Green and gray rubber
Light green plastic
Green
Lavender
Gray

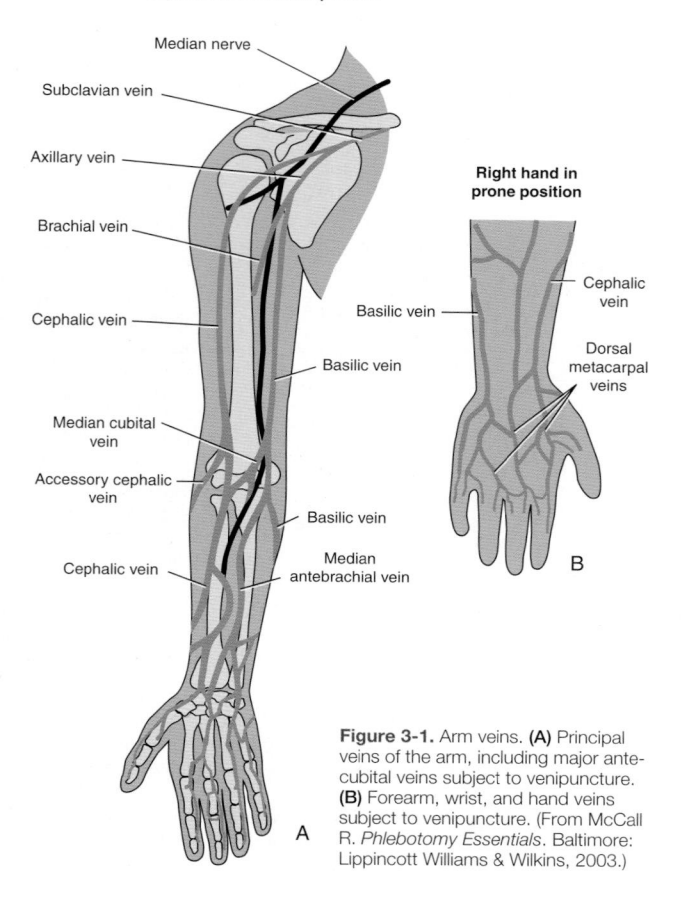

Right arm in anatomic position

Median nerve

Subclavian vein

Axillary vein

Brachial vein

Cephalic vein

Median cubital vein

Accessory cephalic vein

Cephalic vein

Right hand in prone position

Cephalic vein

Basilic vein

Dorsal metacarpal veins

Basilic vein

Basilic vein

Median antebrachial vein

B

Figure 3-1. Arm veins. **(A)** Principal veins of the arm, including major ante-cubital veins subject to venipuncture. **(B)** Forearm, wrist, and hand veins subject to venipuncture. (From McCall R. *Phlebotomy Essentials*. Baltimore: Lippincott Williams & Wilkins, 2003.)

A

TABLE 3-1	Evacuated Tube System: Color Coding	
Tube Color	Additive	Laboratory Use
Purple	Ethylenediaminetetraacetic acid (EDTA)	Hematology testing
Blue	Sodium citrate	Coagulation studies (fill to proper level)
Green	Lithium heparin or sodium heparin	Blood gases and pH; cytogenetics
Gray	Potassium oxalate or sodium fluoride	Glucose testing
Red	None	Serum testing
Red/yellow	Glass particles	Chemistry
Red/gray	Thixotropic gel	Chemistry

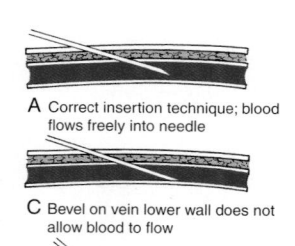

A Correct insertion technique; blood
flows freely into needle

C Bevel on vein lower wall does not
allow blood to flow

E Needle partially inserted and
causes blood leakage into tissue

F When a vein rolls, the needle may
slip to the side of the vein without
penetrating it

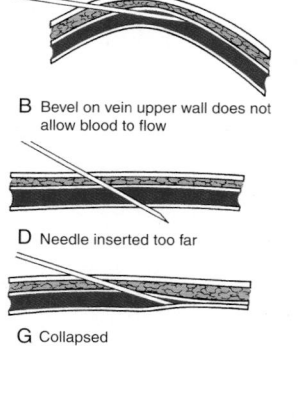

B Bevel on vein upper wall does not
allow blood to flow

D Needle inserted too far

G Collapsed

Figure 3-2. Proper and improper needle positioning. **(A).** Correct needle insertion technique; blood flows freely into tube. **(B).** Bevel on vein upper wall prevents
blood flow. **(C).** Bevel on veing lower wall prevents blood flow. **(D).** Needle
inserted too far penetrates through the vein. **(E).** Partially inserted needle causes
blood leakage into tissue. **(F).** Needle slipped beside the vein, not into it; caused
when a vein rolls to the side. **(G).** Collapsed vein prevents blood flow.

Procedure 3-2 Capillary Puncture

Equipment
- Skin puncture device
- 70% alcohol pads
- 2 × 2 gauze pads
- Microcollection tubes or containers
- Heel-warmer
- Small band-aids
- Pen or permanent marker

1. Double-check the requisition slip.
2. Put on gloves.
3. Select the puncture site (finger or heel) and make sure it is warm (Figs. 3-3 and 3-4).
4. Cleanse the site and allow to air dry.
5. Perform the puncture perpendicular to the whorls of the fingerprint or footprint.
6. Discard puncture device.
7. Wipe away first blood drop with dry gauze.
8. Apply pressure but do not milk the site.
9. Collect the specimen.
10. Cap microcollection tubes; mix additives by gently tilting tubes.
11. Apply clean gauze to the site with pressure; do not apply a dressing to children under age 2.
12. Release the patient when bleeding has stopped.
13. Label the containers.
14. Care for or discard equipment and clean the work area.
15. Remove PPE and wash your hands.
16. Test, transfer, or store the blood specimen according to office policy.
17. Record the procedure.

CHARTING EXAMPLE

07/12/08	OP fingerstick for prothrombin time
9:00 AM	dx ###.## per Dr. Robins.
	———————————————— S. Smith, CMA

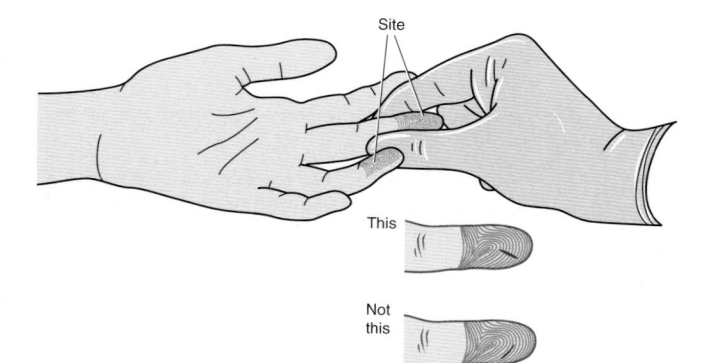

Figure 3-3. Recommend site and direction of finger puncture. (From McCall R. *Phlebotomy Essentials*, 4th ed. Baltimore: Lippincott Williams & Wilkins, 2008.)

HEMATOLOGY

Procedure 3-3 Making a Peripheral Blood Smear

Equipment
- Clean glass slides with frosted ends
- Pencil
- Well-mixed whole blood specimen
- Transfer pipette
- Hand disinfectant
- Surface disinfectant

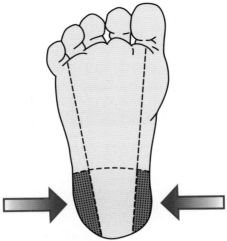

Figure 3-4. Infant heel. Shaded areas indicate safe areas for heel puncture. (From McCall R. *Phlebotomy Essentials*, 4th ed. Baltimore: Lippincott Williams & Wilkins, 2008.)

1. Put on gloves.
2. Obtain an EDTA (lavender-top tube) blood specimen.
3. Place a drop of blood 1 cm from the frosted end of the slide.
4. Place the slide on a flat surface.
5. Hold the spreader slide at a 30-degree angle and draw it back against the blood.

6. Allow blood to spread under the edge, then push spreader slide toward other end.
7. Label the slide on the frosted area.
8. Allow the slide to air dry.
9. Care for or discard equipment and clean the work area.
10. Remove gloves and wash your hands.

Procedure 3-4 Staining a Peripheral Blood Smear

Equipment
- Staining rack
- Wright's stain materials
- Prepared slide
- Tweezers
- Hand disinfectant
- Surface disinfectant

1. Put on gloves, impervious gown, and face shield.
2. Obtain a recently made dried blood smear.
3. Verify that the slide is labeled with correct patient identification.
4. Place the slide on a stain rack blood side up. Place staining solution(s) onto slide according to manufacturer's instructions.
5. Holding the slide with tweezers, gently rinse the slide with water. Wipe off the back of the slide with gauze. Stand the slide upright and allow it to dry.
6. Properly care for or dispose of equipment. Clean the work area.
7. Remove PPE and wash your hands.

Procedure 3-5 Hemoglobin Determination

Equipment
- Hemoglobinometer
- Applicator sticks
- Whole blood
- Hand disinfectant
- Surface disinfectant

1. Put on gloves.
2. Obtain a blood specimen by capillary puncture or use an EDTA (lavender-top tube) blood specimen.
3. Place well-mixed whole blood into the hemoglobinometer chamber.
4. Slide the chamber into the hemoglobinometer.
5. Record the hemoglobin level.
6. Dispose of equipment and clean the work area.
7. Remove gloves and wash your hands.

CHARTING EXAMPLE

12/02/08	Cap puncture L ring finger. HGB 9.5.
10:30 AM	dx code ###.## per Dr. Royal.
	Dr. Royal notified of results.
	——————— R. Smith. CMA

3
Lab

Procedure 3-6   Microhematocrit Determination

Equipment
- Microcollection tubes
- Sealing clay
- Microhematocrit centrifuge
- Microhematocrit reading device
- Hand disinfectant
- Surface disinfectant

 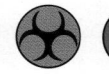 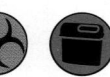

1. Put on gloves.
2. Draw blood into the capillary tube by capillary puncture or from well-mixed EDTA tube of whole blood.
3. Place your forefinger over the tube top.
4. Wipe excess blood off the sides.
5. Push the bottom into sealing clay.
6. Draw a second specimen in the same manner for quality control purposes.
7. Place tubes, clay-sealed end out, in the radial grooves of the microhematocrit centrifuge opposite each other.
8. Put the lid on the grooved area and tighten by turning the knob clockwise.
9. Close the centrifuge lid. Spin for 5 minutes or as directed by the manufacturer.
10. Remove the tubes and read the results. Results should be within 5% of each other; take the average and report as a percentage.
11. Dispose of tubes in a biohazard container.
12. Care for or dispose of other equipment. Clean the work area.
13. Remove gloves and wash your hands.

03/28/08	Capillary puncture, left ring finger.
4:20 PM	Hct: 42%. Dx code ###.## per Dr.
	Erikson. Dr. notified of results.
	_____ M. Mays, CMA

Procedure 3-7 Westergren Erythrocyte Sedimentation Rate

Equipment
- Hand disinfectant
- EDTA blood sample less than 2 hours old
- ESR kit
- Sedimentation rack
- Pipette
- Timer
- Surface disinfectant

1. Put on gloves, impervious gown, and face shield.
2. Verify the patient information on the specimen tube.
3. Gently mix EDTA lavender-stoppered anticoagulation tube for 2 minutes.
4. Using a vial from the ESR kit and a pipette, fill vial to the indicated mark.
5. Replace stopper and invert vial several times to mix.
6. Using an ESR calibrated pipette from the kit, insert the pipette through the tube's stopper with a twist.
7. Push down slowly but firmly until the pipette meets the bottom of the vial.

8. Place the tube in a vertical holder.
9. Wait exactly 1 hour; use a timer for accuracy. Keep the tube straight upright and undisturbed.
10. Record the level of the top of the RBCs after 1 hour. Normal results for men are 0–10 mL/hour; for women, 0–15 mL/hour.
11. Care for or dispose of equipment. Clean the work area.
12. Remove PPE and wash your hands.

URINALYSIS

Procedure 3-8   Clean Catch Midstream Urine Specimen

Equipment
- Sterile urine container labeled with patient's name
- Cleansing towelettes (2 for males, 3 for females)
- Hand sanitizer

1. Put on gloves if you will assist the patient.
2. Provide supplies if the patient is to perform the procedure.
3. Have the patient perform the procedure.
   Instruct male patients to:
   - Expose the glans penis by retracting the foreskin (if uncircumcised), then clean the meatus with an antiseptic wipe.
   - Clean the glans in a circular motion away from the meatus. Use a new wipe for each cleaning sweep.
   - Keeping the foreskin retracted, void a few seconds into the toilet or urinal.
   - Bring the sterile container into the urine stream and collect a sufficient amount (about 30–60 mL).
   - Avoid touching the penis to the inside of the container.
   - Finish voiding into the toilet or urinal.

Instruct female patients to:
- Kneel or squat over a bedpan or toilet bowl.
- Spread the labia minora widely to expose the meatus.
- Use an antiseptic wipe to cleanse on either side of the meatus, then the meatus itself. Use a new wipe for each cleaning sweep.
- Keeping the labia separated, void a few seconds into the toilet.
- Bring the sterile container into the urine stream and collect a sufficient amount (about 30–60 mL).
- Finish voiding into the toilet or bedpan.

4. Cap the filled container and place it in a designated area.
5. Transport the specimen in a biohazard container for testing.
6. Care for or dispose of equipment. Clean the work area.
7. Remove gloves and wash your hands.

Procedure 3-9 24-hour Urine Specimen

Equipment
- Patient's labeled 24-hour urine container (may need more than one)
- Preservatives
- Chemical hazard labels
- Graduated cylinder that holds at least 1 L
- Serological or volumetric pipettes
- Clean random urine container
- Fresh 10% bleach solution
- Hand disinfectant
- Surface disinfectant

1. Identify the type of 24-hour urine collection requested.
2. Check for any special requirements (e.g., addition of acid or preservative).

3. Label the container.
4. Put on gloves, impervious gown, and face shield.
5. Add to the container the correct amount of acid or preservative (if not already included) using a serological or volumetric pipette.
6. Use the provided label or make one with spaces for the patient's name, beginning time and date, and ending time and date.
7. Instruct the patient to collect a 24-hour urine sample:
   • Void into the toilet and note this time and date as beginning.
   • After the first voiding, collect each voiding and add it to the urine container for the next 24 hours.
   • Precisely 24 hours after beginning collection, empty the bladder even if there is no urge to void and add this final volume of urine to the container.
   • Note on the label the ending time and date.
8. Explain that urine may have to be refrigerated the entire time.
9. Have the patient return the specimen when collection is complete.
10. Chart that supplies and instructions were given to collect a 24-hour urine specimen and the test that was requested.
11. When you receive the specimen:
    • Verify beginning and ending times and dates before the patient leaves.
    • Add any acids or preservatives needed before routing the specimen to the testing laboratory.
12. Wearing gloves, impervious gown and face shield, pour the urine into a cylinder to record the volume.
13. Pour an aliquot of the urine into a clean container to be sent to the laboratory. (Label the specimen with the patient's identification.)
14. Record the volume of the urine collection and the amount of any acid or preservative added on the sample container and on the laboratory requisition.
15. If permitted, dispose of the remaining urine.

16. Record the volume on the patient's test requisition and chart.
17. Clean the cylinder with fresh 10% bleach solution, then rinse with water. Let it air dry. For disposable container, place in biohazard container.
18. Clean the work area and dispose of waste.
19. Remove PPE and wash your hands.

WARNING ⚠️

- Use caution when handling acids and other hazardous materials. Be familiar with the material safety data sheets for each chemical in your site.
- Instruct patients not to discard or handle preservative in the container.

Procedure 3-10 Determining Urine Color and Clarity

Equipment
- 10% bleach solution
- Patient's labeled urine specimen
- Clear tube (usually a centrifuge)
- White paper scored with black lines
- Hand disinfectant
- Surface disinfectant

1. Put on gloves and PPE.
2. Verify that the names on the specimen container and report form match.
3. Pour about 10 mL of urine into the tube. If the specimen volume is less that 10 mL, note this on the test result form.

4. In bright light against a white background, examine the color. The most common colors are straw (very pale yellow), yellow, dark yellow, and amber (brown-yellow).
5. Determine clarity. Hold the tube in front of the white paper scored with black lines. If you see the lines clearly (not obscured), record as clear. If you see the lines but they are not well delineated, record as hazy. If you cannot see the lines at all, record as cloudy.
6. Care for or dispose of equipment. Clean the work area.
7. Remove PPE and wash your hands.

CHARTING EXAMPLE

05/31/08 **2:45 PM**	Random urine collected. Yellow/clear. ———————————— H. Henderson, CMA

TABLE 3-2 Causes of Variations in Urine Color and Clarity

Color and Clarity	Possible Causes
Yellow-brown or green brown	Bile in urine (as in jaundice)
Dark yellow or orange	Concentrate urine, low fluid intake, dehydration, inability of kidney to dilute urine, fluorescein (intravenous dye), multivitamins, excessive carotene
Bright orange-red	Pyridium (urinary tract analgesic)
Red or reddish-brown	Hemoglobin pigments, pyrvinium pamoate (Povan) for intestinal worms, sulfonamides (sulfa-based antibiotics)
Green or blue	Artificial color in food or drugs
Blackish, grayish, smoky	Hemoglobin or remnants of old red blood cells (indicating bleeding in upper urinary tract, chyle, prostatic fluid, yeasts)
Cloudy	Phosphate precipitation (normal after sitting for a long time), urates (compound of uric acid), leukocytes, pus, blood, epithelial cells, fat droplets, strict vegetarian diet

3
Lab

Procedure 3-11 Chemical Reagent Strip Analysis

Equipment
- Patient's labeled urine specimen
- Chemical strip (such as Multistix or Chemstrip)
- Manufacturer's color comparison chart
- Stopwatch or timer
- Hand disinfectant
- Surface disinfectant

1. Put on gloves and PPE.
2. Verify the names on the specimen container and report form match.
3. Mix the patient's urine by gently swirling the covered container.
4. Remove the reagent strip from its container and replace the lid.
5. Immerse the reagent strip completely in the urine then immediately remove it. Slide the strip edge along the container's lip to remove excess urine.
6. Start stopwatch or timer immediately.
7. Compare the reagent pads to the color chart, determining results at the intervals stated by the manufacturer.
8. Read all reactions at the times indicated and record the results.
9. Discard the reagent strips in the proper receptacle. Discard urine unless more testing is required.
10. Clean the work area.
11. Remove PPE and wash your hands.

Procedure 3-12 Preparing Urine Sediment

Equipment
- Patient's labeled urine specimen
- Urine centrifuge tubes
- Transfer pipette
- Centrifuge (1,500–2,000 rpm)
- Hand disinfectant
- Surface disinfectant

1. Put on gloves and PPE.
2. Verify the names on the specimen container and report form match.
3. Swirl specimen to mix. Pour 10 mL of well-mixed urine into a labeled centrifuge tube or standard system tube and cap with a plastic cap or parafilm.
4. Centrifuge the sample at 1,500 rpm for 5 minutes.
5. Remove the tubes when the centrifuge has stopped.
6. Make sure no tests are to be performed first on the supernatant.
7. Remove the caps and pour off the supernatant, leaving 0.5–1.0 mL. Suspend the sediment again by aspirating up and down with a transfer pipette, or follow manufacturer's directions.
8. Care for and dispose of equipment. Clean the work area.
9. Remove PPE and wash your hands.

SPECIMEN COLLECTION AND MICROBIOLOGY

> **BOX 3-2** Guidelines for Specimen Collection and Handling
>
> - Follow the CDC's standard precautions for specimen collection.
> - Review requirements for collecting and handling the specimen, including equipment, specimen type to be collected, amount required for laboratory analysis, and handling and storage procedure.
> - Use only the appropriate specimen container as specified by the medical office or laboratory.
> - Ensure that the specimen container is sterile to prevent contamination by organisms not present at the collection site.
> - Examine each container before use to make sure that it is not damaged, the medium is intact and moist, and it is well within the expiration date.
> - Label each tube or specimen container with the patient's name and/or identification number, the date, the name or initials of the person collecting the specimen, the specimen source or site, and any other required information.

Procedure 3-13 Collecting a Throat Specimen

Equipment
- Tongue blade
- Light source
- Sterile specimen container and swab
- Hand sanitizer
- Surface sanitizer
- Biohazard transport bag (if to be sent to the laboratory for analysis)

1. Put on PPE.
2. Have the patient sit with a light source directed in the throat.
3. Remove the sterile swab from the container. If performing both the rapid strep and culture or confirming negative results with a culture, swab with two swabs held together.
4. Have the patient say "Ah" as you press down with the tongue depressor.
5. Swab the mucous membranes, especially the tonsillar area, the crypts, and the posterior pharynx in a "figure 8" motion. Turn the swab to expose all of its surfaces to the membranes. Avoid touching tongue, teeth, sides of mouth, and uvula.
6. Withdraw the swab with tongue depressor still in position.
7. Follow the instructions on the specimen container for transferring the swab or processing the specimen in the office using a commercial kit.
8. Label the specimen with the patient's name, collection date and time, and the material's origin.
9. Dispose of supplies in a biohazard waste container.
10. Remove PPE and wash your hands.
11. Route the specimen or store it until routing can be completed.
12. Document the procedure.
13. Sanitize the work area.

CHARTING EXAMPLE

11/20/08 10:30 AM	Throat specimen obtained, Dx code ###.## per Dr. Lewis. Rapid strep test negative, specimen to reference lab for C&S.
	———————— M. Mohr, CMA

3
Lab

Procedure 3-14 Collecting a Nasopharyngeal Specimen

Equipment
- Penlight
- Tongue blade
- Sterile flexible wire swab
- Transport media
- Hand sanitizer
- Surface sanitizer
- Biohazard transport bag (if specimen will be sent to the laboratory for analysis)

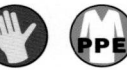

1. Put on gloves and PPE.
2. Have patient tilt the head back.
3. Inspect the nasopharyngeal area using a penlight and tongue blade.
4. Gently swab through the nostril and into the nasopharynx, keeping the swab near the septum and floor of the nose. Rotate the swab quickly, remove it, and place it in the transport media. Avoid touching the sides of the patient's nostril or tongue to prevent specimen contamination.
5. Label the specimen with the patient's name, collection date and time, and the specimen's origin.
6. Dispose of equipment in a biohazard waste container.
7. Remove PPE and wash your hands.
8. Route the specimen or store it until routing can be completed.
9. Document the procedure.
10. Sanitize the work area.

11/20/08	Nasopharyngeal specimen obtained,
10:30 AM	Dx code ###.## per Dr. Lewis.
	Specimen to reference lab for C&S.
	———————————— M. Mohr, CMA

Procedure 3-15 Collecting a Wound Specimen

Equipment
- Sterile swab
- Transport media
- Hand sanitizer
- Surface sanitizer
- Biohazard transport bag (if specimen will be sent to the laboratory for analysis)

1. Put on PPE.
2. If dressing is present, remove it and dispose of it in biohazard container.
3. Assess the wound by observing color, odor, and exudate amount.
4. Remove contaminated gloves and put on clean gloves.
5. Use the sterile swab to sample the exudate. Saturate swab with exudate, avoiding the skin edge around the wound.
6. Place swab in container and crush ampule of transport medium.
7. Label the specimen with the patient's name, collection date and time, and the specimen's origin.

71

8. Route the specimen or store it until routing can be completed.
9. Clean the wound and apply a sterile dressing.
10. Dispose of equipment in a biohazard waste container.
11. Remove PPE and wash your hands.
12. Document the procedure.
13. Sanitize the work area.

CHARTING EXAMPLE

11/20/08 **10:30 AM**	Wound specimen obtained from right heel, Dx code ###.## per Dr. Lewis. Specimen to reference lab for C&S. ———————— M. Mohr, CMA

Procedure 3-16 Collecting a Sputum Specimen

Equipment
- Sterile specimen container
- Hand sanitizer
- Surface sanitizer
- Biohazard transport bag

1. Put on PPE.
2. Have the patient rinse mouth with water.
3. Have the patient cough deeply.

4. Have the patient expectorate directly into the specimen container. About 5 to 10 mL is sufficient for most sputum studies.
5. Handle the specimen container according to standard precautions. Cap the container immediately and put it into the biohazard bag for transport to the laboratory. Fill out a laboratory requisition slip to accompany the specimen.
6. Label the specimen with the patient's name, collection date and time, and the specimen's origin.
7. Route the specimen to the laboratory.
8. Dispose of equipment in a biohazard waste container.
9. Remove PPE and wash your hands.
10. Document the procedure.
11. Sanitize the work area.

CHARTING EXAMPLE

11/20/08	Moderate amount of thick, yellow sputum,
10:30 AM	Dx code ###.## per Dr. Lewis.
	Specimen to reference lab for C&S.
	———————— M. Mohr, CMA

Procedure 3-17 Collecting a Stool Specimen

Equipment
- Specimen container (depends on test ordered)
- Test kit or slide for occult blood testing
- Tongue blade or wooden spatula
- Hand sanitizer
- Surface sanitizer
- Biohazard transport bag

1. Explain any dietary, medication, or other restrictions necessary for the collection.
2. Instruct patient to defecate into a disposable plastic container or onto plastic wrap placed over the toilet bowl. When obtaining a stool specimen for C&S or ova and parasites, instruct the patient to collect a small amount of the first and last portion of the stool after the bowel movement with the wooden spatula or tongue blade and place it in the specimen container without contaminating the outside of the container. Fill Para-Pak until fluid reaches "fill" line and recap the container.
3. Upon receiving the specimen, put on gloves and place specimen in biohazard bag for transport to the reference laboratory.
4. Fill out a laboratory requisition slip.
5. Label the specimen with the patient's name, collection date and time, and the specimen's origin.
6. Transport the specimen to the laboratory or store as directed.
7. Properly dispose of equipment in a biohazard waste container.
8. Remove PPE and wash your hands.
9. Document the procedure, including patient instructions.
10. Sanitize the work area.

11/20/08	Patient instructed on preparation for and
10:30 AM	collection of stool for occult blood. Patient
	demonstrated understanding and will
	return specimen to lab upon completion.
	Dx code ###.## per Dr. Lewis.
	——————————— M. Mohr, CMA

11/21/08	Patient delivered stool specimen to the
8:00 AM	laboratory.
	——————————— M. Mohr, CMA

BOX 3-3 Special Stool Specimens

Follow these tips when collecting stool specimens to test for pinworms or parasites or to obtain a swab for culture. Remember to follow standard precautions.

- *Pinworms:* Schedule the appointment early in the morning, preferably before a bowel movement or bath. Pinworms tend to leave the rectum and lay eggs around the anus during the night. Press clear adhesive tape against the anal area. Remove it quickly and place it sticky side down on a glass slide for the physician to inspect.
- *Parasites:* Caution the patient not to use a laxative or enema before the test to avoid destroying the evidence of parasites. If the stool contains blood or mucus, include as much as possible in the specimen container, because these substances are most likely to contain the suspected organism.
- *Stool culture:* A sterile cotton-tipped swab is passed into the rectal canal beyond the sphincter and rotated carefully. Place it in the appropriate culture container or process as directed for smear preparation.

Procedure 3-18 Testing Stool Specimen for Occult Blood

Equipment
- Patient's labeled specimen pack
- Developer or reagent drops
- Hand sanitizer
- Surface sanitizer
- Contaminated waste container

1. Put on gloves.
2. Verify identification on the patient's prepared test pack.
3. Check expiration date for developing solution.
4. Open the test window on the back of the pack and apply one drop of the developer or testing reagent to each window according to manufacturer's directions. Read the color change within the specified time, usually 60 seconds.
5. Apply one drop of developer as directed on the control monitor section or window of the pack. Note whether the quality control results are positive or negative. If results are acceptable, report patient results. If results are not acceptable, notify physician.
6. Dispose of the test pack and gloves. Wash your hands.
7. Record the procedure.
8. Sanitize the work area.

03/28/08 3:00 PM	Occult blood slides ×3 returned to office via mail; testing performed. Dx ###.## per Dr. Franklin; findings positive. Dr. Franklin notified.
	———————————— J. Smith, RMA

Procedure 3-19 Collecting Blood for Culture

Equipment
- Specimen container (depends on testing site; yellow-top sodium polyanethol sulfonate vacutainer tubes or aerobic and anaerobic blood culture bottles)
- Blood culture skin prep packs (or 70% isopropyl alcohol wipes and povidone-iodine solution swabs or towelettes)
- Venipuncture supplies
- Hand sanitizer
- Surface sanitizer

1. Check expiration dates for supplies.
2. Put on PPE.
3. Verify that the patient has not started antibiotic therapy. If therapy has started, document antibiotic, strength, dose, duration, and time of last dose.
4. Prepare the site:
   - Apply alcohol to venipuncture site and allow to air dry.
   - Apply povidone-iodine prep in progressively increasing concentric circles without wiping back over skin that is already prepped.

77

- Let stand at least one minute and allow to air dry. Do not touch skin.
- Swab the antecubital space using a povidone-iodine swab, cleaning in progressively increasing circles.
5. Wipe bottle stoppers with povidone-iodine solution.
6. Perform venipuncture (Procedure 3-1).
7. Fill bottles or tube. Invert each 8 to 10 times as soon as collected. If using culture bottles, fill the aerobic bottle first.
8. Complete venipuncture.
9. Use an isopropyl alcohol wipe to remove residual povidone-iodine from skin.
10. Label the specimen with the patient's name, the collection date and time, and the specimen's origin.
11. Remove gloves and wash hands.
12. In preparation for the second collection 30 minutes after the first, put on new gloves and repeat steps 4 to 10 at a second venipuncture site.
13. Dispose of the equipment in a biohazard waste container.
14. Remove PPE and wash your hands.
15. Document the procedure.
16. Sanitize the work area.

CHARTING EXAMPLE

11/20/08	Blood culture specimens collected from
10:30 AM	antecubital area of left and right arms,
	Dx code ###.## per Dr. Lewis.
	—————————— M. Mohr, CMA

Procedure 3-20 Collecting Genital Specimens for Culture

Equipment
- Specimen container (depends on testing requested; bacterial, viral, and Chlamydia specimens require different media)
- Hand sanitizer
- Surface sanitizer

1. Check expiration dates for supplies.
2. Put on PPE.
3. Verbally verify patient identification.
4. Accept specimens from the physician; secure them in the appropriate medium and follow instructions for that particular medium.
5. Label the specimen with the patient's name, collection date and time, and the specimen's origin.
6. Repeat steps 4 and 5 for each specimen.
7. Store specimens appropriately until transport.
8. Dispose of equipment in biohazard waste container.
9. Remove PPE and wash your hands.
10. Document the procedure.
11. Sanitize the work area.

CHARTING EXAMPLE

11/20/08 10:30 AM	Vaginal specimens collected for C&S, herpes, and Chlamydia and referred to reference lab, Dx code ###.## per Dr. Lewis.
	———————— M. Mohr, CMA

TABLE 3-3 Handling and Storing Commonly Collected Specimens

	Handling	Storage
Urine	Clean-catch midstream with care to avoid contaminating the inside of the container; must not stand more than 1 hour after collection.	Refrigerate if cannot be tested within 1 hour; add preservative at direction of laboratory; preservatives not usually used for urine culture.
Blood	Handle carefully, as hemolysis may destroy microorganisms; collect in anticoagulant tube at room temperature; specimen must remain free of contaminants; see laboratory manual for proper anticoagulant.	For most specimens, refrigerate at 4°C (39°F) to slow changes in physical and chemical composition.
Stool	Collect in clean container. To test for ova and parasites, keep warm.	Deliver to laboratory immediately. If delayed, mix with preservative provided or recommended by laboratory, or use transport medium.
Microbiology specimens	Do not contaminate swab or inside of specimen container by touching either to surface other than site of collection. Protect anaerobic specimens from exposure to air.	Transport specimen as soon as possible. If delayed, refrigerate at 4°C (39°F) to maintain integrity.

Observe standard precautions while handling any of these specimens.

TABLE **3-4**	Categorizing Bacteria
Morphology	Types
Round (spherical)	Cocci
Grapelike clusters	Staphylococci
Chain formations	Streptococci
Paired	Diplococci
Rod-shaped	Bacilli
Somewhat oval	Coccobacilli
End-to-end chains	Streptobacilli
Spiral	Spirochetes
Flexible (usually with flagella, whiplike extremities that aid movement)	Spirilla
Rigid, curved rods (comma-shaped)	Vibrios

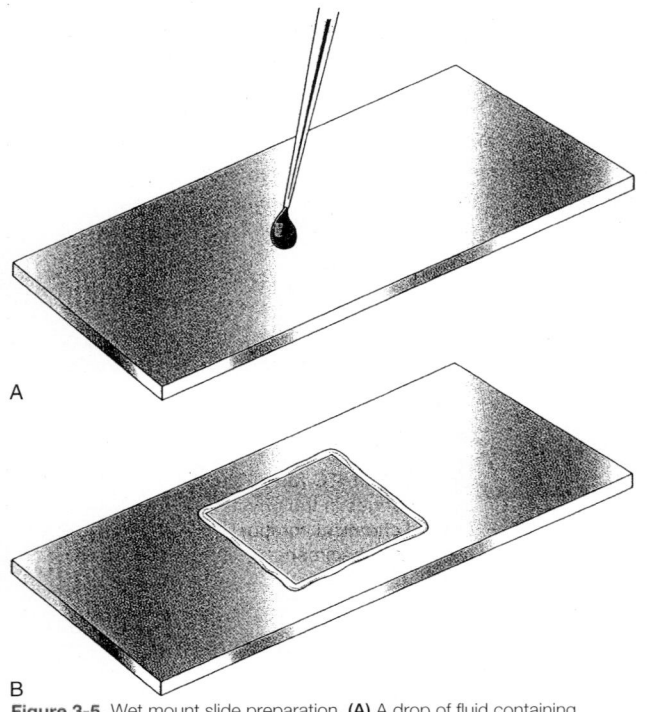

A

B

Figure 3-5. Wet mount slide preparation. **(A)** A drop of fluid containing the organism is placed on a glass slide. **(B)** The specimen is covered with a coverslip ringed with petroleum jelly.

Procedure 3-21 Preparing a Smear for Microscopic Evaluation

Equipment
- Specimen
- Bunsen burner
- Slide forceps
- Slide
- Sterile swab or inoculating loop
- Pencil or diamond-tipped pen
- Hand sanitizer
- Surface sanitizer

1. Label the slide with patient identification.
2. Put on PPE.
3. Hold the edges of the slide between the thumb and index finger. Starting at the right side of the slide, spread the material from the specimen over the slide to thinly fill the center of the slide. Do not rub the material vigorously over the slide.
4. Dispose of the contaminated swab or disposable inoculating loop in a biohazard container.
5. Allow the smear to air dry in a flat position for at least half an hour. Do not blow on the slide or wave it about in the air. Do not apply heat until the specimen has dried. Some specimens (e.g., Pap smear) require a fixative spray.
6. Hold the dried smear slide with the forceps. Pass the slide quickly through the flame of a lighter or safety match three or four times. The slide has been fixed properly when the back of the slide feels slightly uncomfortably warm to the back of the gloved hand. It should not feel hot. *Caution:* Any excess heat will distort and probably destroy the specimen material on the slide.
7. Dispose of the equipment in a biohazard waste container.

8. Remove PPE and wash your hands.
9. Document the procedure.
10. Sanitize the work area.

Procedure 3-22   Performing a Gram Stain

Equipment
- Crystal violet stain
- Staining rack
- Gram iodine solution
- Wash bottle with distilled water
- Alcohol-acetone solution
- Counterstain (e.g., Safranin)
- Absorbent (bibulous) paper pad
- Labeled specimen on glass slide (see Procedure 3-21)
- Bunsen burner
- Slide forceps
- Stopwatch or timer
- Hand sanitizer
- Surface sanitizer

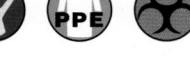

1. Ensure the specimen is heat-fixed to the labeled slide and the slide is room temperature.
2. Put on PPE.
3. Place slide smear side up on staining rack.
4. Flood the smear with crystal violet. Time for 60 seconds.
5. Using forceps, tilt the slide about 45 degrees to drain excess dye then rinse with distilled water about 5 seconds; drain excess water.
6. Replace slide on rack. Flood with Gram iodine solution for 60 seconds.
7. Using forceps, tilt the slide 45 degrees to drain iodine solution then rinse with distilled water from the wash bottle for about 5 to 10 seconds.

8. Wash the slide with the alcohol-acetone solution until no more stain runs off.
9. Rinse slide with distilled water for 5 seconds and return to the rack.
10. Flood with Safranin or suitable counterstain for 60 seconds.
11. Drain excess counterstain from the slide by tilting it 45 degrees, then rinse with distilled water for 5 seconds to remove the counterstain.
12. Gently blot the smear dry with bibulous paper. Do not disturb the smeared specimen.
13. Wipe the back of the slide clear of any solution. Place between the pages of a bibulous paper pad and gently press to remove excess moisture, if needed.
14. Dispose of equipment in a biohazard waste container.
15. Remove PPE and wash your hands.
16. Document the procedure.
17. Sanitize the work area.

Procedure 3-23   Inoculating a Culture

Equipment
- Specimen on a swab or loop
- China marker or permanent laboratory marker
- Sterile or disposable loop
- Bunsen burner
- Labeled Petri dish
- Hand sanitizer
- Surface sanitizer

1. Put on PPE.
2. Label the medium side of the plate with the patient's name, identification number, source of specimen, time collected, time inoculated, your initials, and date.
3. Remove the Petri plate from the cover and place the cover on the work surface with the opening up.
4. Streak the specimen swab clear across half of the plate, starting at the top and working to the center. Dispose of the swab in a biohazard container.
5. Use a disposable loop.
6. Turn the plate a quarter-turn. Pass the loop a few times in the original inoculum then across the medium approximately a quarter of the surface of the plate. Do not enter the originally streaked area after the first few sweeps.
7. Turn the plate another quarter-turn so that now it is 180 degrees to the original smear. Draw the loop at right angles through the most recently streaked area. Again, do not enter the originally streaked area after the first few sweeps.
8. Dispose of equipment in a biohazard waste container.
9. Remove PPE and wash your hands.
10. Document the procedure.
11. Sanitize the work area.

IMMUNOLOGY

Procedure 3-24 Mono Testing

Equipment
- Patient's labeled specimen
- CLIA-waived mononucleosis kit (slide or test strip)
- Stopwatch or timer
- Hand sanitizer
- Surface sanitizer

1. Verify that the names on the specimen container and the laboratory form match.
2. Ensure that materials in the kit and the patient specimen are at room temperature.
3. Label the test pack or test strip (depending on type of kit) with the patient's name, positive control, and negative control. Use one test pack or strip per patient and control.
4. Aspirate the patient's specimen using the transfer pipette and place volume indicated in kit package insert on the sample well of the test pack or dip test strip labeled with the patient's name.
5. Sample the positive and negative controls as directed in step 4.
6. Set timer for incubation period indicated in package insert.
7. Read reaction results at the end of incubation period.
8. Verify the results of the controls before documenting the patient's results. Log controls and patient information on the worksheet.
9. Dispose of equipment in a biohazard waste container.
10. Remove PPE and wash your hands.
11. Document the procedure.
12. Sanitize the work area.

CHARTING EXAMPLE

04/23/08	Mono test performed, Dx code ###.##
10:00 AM	per Dr. Scott. Results negative.

——————————— S. Miller, CMA

Procedure 3-25 HCG Pregnancy Test

Equipment
- Patient's labeled specimen
- HCG pregnancy kit (test pack and transfer pipettes or test strip; kit contents will vary by manufacturer)
- HCG positive and negative control (different controls may be needed when testing urine)
- Timer
- Hand sanitizer
- Surface sanitizer

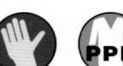

1. Verify that the names on the specimen container and the laboratory form match.
2. Label the test pack or strip (depending on type of kit) with the patient's name, positive control, and negative control. Use one test pack or strip per patient and control.
3. Note in the patient's information and in the control log whether you are using urine, plasma, or serum. Be sure that the kit and controls are at room temperature.
4. Aspirate the patient's specimen using the transfer pipette and place volume indicated in kit package insert on the sample well of the test pack or dip test strip labeled with the patient's name.
5. Sample the positive and negative controls as directed in step 4.
6. Set timer for incubation period indicated in package insert.
7. Read reaction results at the end of incubation period.
8. Verify the results of the controls before documenting the patient's results. Log controls and patient information on the worksheet.
9. Dispose of equipment in a biohazard waste container.
10. Remove PPE and wash your hands.
11. Document the procedure.
12. Sanitize the work area.

| 12/14/08 10:00 AM | HCG test performed on urine, Dx code ###.## per Dr. Schanzer. Positive result reported to doctor. |

———————— J. Simpson, CMA

Procedure 3-26 Rapid Group A Strep Testing

Equipment
- Patient's labeled throat specimen
- Group A strep kit
- Timer
- Hand sanitizer
- Surface sanitizer

1. Verify that the names on the specimen container and the laboratory form match.
2. Label one extraction tube with the patient's name, one for the positive control, and one for the negative control.
3. Follow the directions for the kit. Add the appropriate reagents and drops to each of the extraction tubes. Avoid splashing, and use the correct number of drops.
4. Insert the patient's swab into the labeled extraction tube.
5. Add the appropriate controls to each of the labeled extraction tubes.
6. Set the timer for the appropriate time to ensure accuracy.
7. Add the appropriate reagent and drops to each of the extraction tubes.

8. Use the swab to mix the reagents. Then press out any excess fluid on the swab against the inside of the tube.
9. Add three drops from the well-mixed extraction tube to the sample window of the strep A test unit or dip the test stick labeled with the patient's name. Do the same for each control.
10. Set the timer for the time indicated in the kit package insert.
11. A positive result appears as a line in the result window within 5 minutes. The strep A test unit or strip has an internal control; if a line appears in the control window, the test is valid.
12. Read a negative result at exactly 5 minutes to avoid a false negative.
13. Verify results of the controls before recording or reporting test results. Log the controls and the patient's information on the worksheet.
14. Dispose of equipment in a biohazard waste container.
15. Remove PPE and wash your hands.
16. Document the procedure.
17. Sanitize the work area.

CHARTING EXAMPLE

05/22/08 11:15 AM	Group A rapid strep test performed, dx code ###.## per Dr. Harrison. Positive result reported to physician.
	——————————— B. White, CMA

BOX 3-5 Tips and Troubleshooting for Immunoassays

1. Follow the times exactly.
2. Add reagents in correct order.
3. Use reagents only with other reagents from the same kit.
4. Use exact amount of reagents stated in directions.
5. Ensure that reagents and samples are at room temperature.
6. Ensure that reagents have not expired.

If an immunoassay control is not producing an acceptable result, try the following:

1. Reread the procedure to be sure a step was not omitted.
2. Check the labels of reagents to be sure the correct reagents were added in the correct order.
3. Visually check reagents for signs of contamination, such as cloudiness or color change.
4. Repeat the test with a new bottle of control.
5. Repeat the test with a new kit or reagent.
6. Call the manufacturer for assistance.

CHEMISTRY TESTING

Procedure 3-27 Blood Glucose Testing

Equipment
- Glucose meter
- Glucose reagent strips
- Control solutions
- Capillary puncture device
- Alcohol pad
- Gauze
- Paper towel
- Adhesive bandage
- Hand sanitizer
- Surface sanitizer

1. Review instrument manual for your glucose meter.
2. Turn on glucose meter and ensure calibration.
3. Perform the test on the quality control material. Record results. Determine whether QC is within control limits. If yes, proceed. If no, take corrective action and recheck controls. Document corrective action. Proceed with patient testing when acceptable QC results are obtained.
4. Remove one reagent strip, lay it on the paper towel, and recap the container.
5. Have the patient wash hands in warm water.
6. Cleanse the selected puncture site (finger) with alcohol.
7. Perform a capillary puncture. Wipe away the first drop of blood.
8. Turn the patient's hand palm down and gently squeeze the finger to form a large drop of blood.
9. Bring the reagent strip up to the finger and touch the pad to the blood. Do not touch the finger. Completely cover the pad or fill the testing chamber with blood.
10. Insert reagent strip into analyzer and apply pressure to the puncture wound with gauze.
11. Record the reading from the instrument display.
12. Apply bandage to the patient's fingertip.
13. Dispose of equipment in biohazard container. Clean the work area.
14. Remove PPE and wash your hands.

02/12/08	Capillary puncture left middle finger for
10:00 AM	glucose, dx ###.## per Dr. Miller. Glucose
	tested with meter. Results: 60 mg/dL.
	Dr. Peters notified.
	———————————— M. Miller, CMA

Procedure 3-28 Blood Cholesterol Testing

Equipment
- Cholesterol meter and supplies or test kit
- Control solutions
- Capillary puncture equipment or blood specimen
- Hand sanitizer
- Surface sanitizer

1. Review instrument manual for your cholesterol meter or kit.
2. Perform the test on the quality control material. Record results. Determine whether QC is within control limits. If yes, proceed. If no, take corrective action and recheck controls. Document corrective action. Proceed with patient testing when acceptable QC results are obtained.

3
Lab

3. Follow manufacturer's instructions in using a patient specimen obtained by capillary puncture or from vacutainer tube.
4. Follow manufacturer's instructions for applying the sample to the testing device and inserting the device into the analyzer. Record results.
5. Dispose of equipment in biohazard container. Clean the work area.
6. Remove PPE and wash your hands.

CHARTING EXAMPLE

02/12/08	Cholesterol test performed. Dx ###.##
10:00 AM	per Dr. Peters. Results: 274 mg/dL.
	Dr. Peters notified.
	—————————— M. Miller, CMA

TABLE 3-5	Lab Tests and Normal Values

TABLE 3-5A	Routine Urinalysis

Test	Normal Value
General characteristics and measurements	
Color	Pale yellow to amber
Appearance (clarity)	Clear to slightly hazy
Specific gravity	1.003–1.030
pH	5.0–8.0
Chemical determinations	
Glucose	Negative
Ketones	Negative
Protein	Negative
Bilirubin	Negative
Urobilinogen	0.2–1.0 Ehrlich units/dL
Blood (occult)	Negative
Nitrite	Negative

TABLE **3-5B**	Complete Blood Count (CBC)
Test	Normal Value*
Red blood cell (RBC) count	Men: 4.6–6.2 million/μL Women: 4.2–5.4 million/μL
Hemoglobin (Hb)	Men: 13–18 g/dL Women: 12–16 g/dL
Hematocrit (Hct) or packed cell volume (PCV)	Men: 45%–52% Women: 37%–48%
Red blood cell (RBC) indices (examples)	
Mean corpuscular volume (MCV)	80–95 μL/red cell
Mean corpuscular hemoglobin (MCH)	27–31 pg/red cell
Mean corpuscular hemoglobin concentration (MCHC)	32–36 g/dL
White blood cell (WBC) count	4,300–10,800 μL
Platelets	200,000–400,000/μL

*Values vary depending on instrumentation and type of test.

TABLE 3-5C	Blood Chemistry Tests
Test	Normal Value
Basic panel: An overview of electrolytes, waste product management, and metabolism	
Blood urea nitrogen (BUN)	7–18 mg/dL
Carbon dioxide (CO_2) (includes bicarbonate)	22–29 mmol/L
Chloride (Cl)	98–107 mmol/L
Creatinine	0.5–1.2 mg/dL
Glucose	Fasting: 70–100 mg/dL Random: 85–125 mg/dL
Potassium (K)	3.4–5.0 mmol/L
Sodium (Na)	135–145 mmol/L
Additional blood chemistry tests	
Alanine aminotransferase (ALT)	6–47* U/L
Albumin	2.5–5.7 g/dL
Alkaline phosphatase (ALP)	30–95 U/L*
Amylase	<180 U/L*
Aspartate aminotransferase (AST)	5–30 U/L*

TABLE 3-5C	Blood Chemistry Tests *(Continued)*
Test	**Normal Value**
Bilirubin, total	<1.5 mg/dL
Calcium (Ca)	8.6–10.0 mg/dL
Cholesterol	<200 mg/dL
Creatine phosphokinase (CPK or CK)	130–250 U/L*
Iron, serum (Fe)	40–60 µg/dL
High-density lipoproteins (HDLs)	>40 mg/dL
Lactic dehydrogenase (LDH or LD)	95–200 U/L*
Lipase	<60 U/L*
Low-density lipoproteins (LDLs)	<130 mg/dL
Magnesium (Mg)	1.2–2.1 mEq/L
Phosphorus ((Page*)) (inorganic)	2.7–4.5 mg/dL
Protein, total	6–8 g/dL
Thyroxin (T$_4$)	4.0–12.0 µg/dL (may vary by test method)

TABLE 3-5C	Blood Chemistry Tests (*Continued*)
Test	Normal Value
Thyroid-stimulating hormone (TSH)	0.5–5.0 mIU/L
Triglycerides	<150 mg/dL
Uric acid	Men: 3.5–7.2 mg/dL Women: 2.6–6.0 mg/dL

*Varies significantly by test method.
Compare patient results to normal range printed on laboratory report.
Adapted from Memmler RL, Cohen BJ, Wood DL. *The Human Body in Health and Disease*, 10th ed. Baltimore: Lippincott Williams & Wilkins, 2005.

TABLE **3-6**	Routine Radiographic Examinations by Body Region
Region	Patient Preparation
Trunk	Disrobing of the area: chest, ribs, sternum, shoulder, scapula, clavicle, abdomen, hip, pelvis, and sternoclavicular, acromioclavicular, sacroiliac joints
Extremities	Removing jewelry or clothing that might obscure parts of interest: fingers, thumb, hand, wrist, forearm, elbow, humerus, toes, foot, os calcis, ankle, lower leg, knee, patella, femur
Spine	Disrobing of the appropriate area: cervical, thoracic, or lumbar spine; sacrum; coccyx
Head	Removing eyewear, false eyes, false teeth, earrings, hairpins, hairpieces; skull, sinuses, nasal bones, facial bones and orbits, optic foramen, mandible, temporomandibular joints, mastoid and petrous portion, zygomatic arch

Medication Administration

4

BOX 4-1 **Converting Measurements**

Converting Apothecary or Household to Metric:
* To change ounces (household) to milliliters (metric system), multiply the ounces by 30. Example: 4 oz × 30 = 120 mL.
* To change kilograms (metric system) to pounds (household system), multiply the kilograms by 2.2. Example: 50 kg × 2.2 = 110.0 lb.
* To change pounds to kilograms (metric system), divide the pounds (household system) by 2.2. Example: 44 lb ÷ 2.2 = 20 kg.

Converting Metric to Metric:
* To change grams to milligrams, multiply grams by 1000 or move the decimal point three places to the right. Example: 0.5 grams × 1000 = 500 mg
* To change milligrams to grams, divide the milligrams by 1000 or move the decimal point three places to the left. Example: 500 mg ÷ 1000 = 0.5 g.
* To change liters to milliliters, multiply the liters by 1000 or move the decimal three places to the right. Example: 0.01 L × 1000 = 10 mL.
* To change milliliters to liters, divide the milliliters by 1000 or move the decimal three places to the left. Example: 100 mL ÷ 1000 = 0.1 L.

(No conversion is necessary when changing cubic centimeters to milliliters; they are approximately the same.)

TABLE 4-1 Commonly Prescribed Medications

The following alphabetical list of commonly prescribed drugs (trade and generic) is based on listings of prescriptions dispensed in the United States during 2005. The classification and major therapeutic uses for each are also provided. Trade-name drugs begin with a capital letter; the generic names accompany them in parentheses. All generic names are set in lowercase.

Name	Classification	Major Therapeutic Uses
acetaminophen and codeine	NSAID (analgesic/antipyretic) and opiate (narcotic) combination	moderate to severe pain, fever
AcipHex (rabeprazole)	PPI (gastric acid secretion inhibitor)	PUD, GERD
Actonel (risedronate)	bisphosphonate (bone resorption inhibitor)	osteoporosis; Paget disease
Actos (pioglitazone)	oral antidiabetic	type 2 DM
acyclovir	antiviral	viral infections

TABLE 4-1	Commonly Prescribed Medications (*Continued*)	
Name	Classification	Major Therapeutic Uses
Adderall XR (amphetamine mixed salts)	CNS stimulant	ADHD
Advair Diskus (salmeterol and fluticasone)	adrenergic agonist (bronchodilator); glucocorticoid (anti-inflammatory)	asthma
albuterol aerosol	adrenergic agonist (bronchodilator)	asthma, bronchitis
Allegra (fexofenadine)	antihistamine	allergy
alprazolam	benzodiazepine (anxiolytic, sedative, hypnotic)	anxiety
Altace (ramipril)	ACE inhibitor	hypertension, CHF
Amaryl (glimepiride)	oral antidiabetic	type 2 DM

TABLE 4-1	Commonly Prescribed Medications (Continued)	
Name	Classification	Major Therapeutic Uses
Ambien (zolpidem)	sedative; hypnotic	insomnia
amoxicillin	penicillin (antibiotic)	bacterial infections
Aricept (donepezil)	acetylcholinesterase inhibitor	Alzheimer disease
atenolol	cardioselective β-blocker (antihypertensive, antiarrhythmic, antianginal)	hypertension, angina pectoris, cardiac arrhythmias
Augmentin (amoxicillin and clavulanate)	penicillin (antibiotic) and β-lactamase inhibitor combination	bacterial infections
Avandia (rosiglitazone)	oral antidiabetic	type 2 DM
Aviane (levonorgestrel and ethinyl estradiol)	oral contraceptive	birth control
azithromycin	macrolide (antibiotic)	bacterial infections

Name	Classification	Major Therapeutic Uses
Biaxin (clarithromycin)	macrolide (antibiotic)	bacterial infections
Bupropion SR	atypical antide pressant	depression
buspirone	anxiolytic	anxiety
Celebrex (celecoxib)	Cox-2 inhibitor (NSAID)	pain, inflammation, fever, arthritis
cephalexin	cephalosporin (antibiotic)	bacterial infections
Cialis (tadalafil)	phosphodiesterase (type 5) enzyme inhibitor	ED
ciprofloxacin	fluoroquinolone (antibiotic)	bacterial infections
Clarinex (desloratadine)	antihistamine	allergy
clindamycin	antibiotic	bacterial infections

TABLE 4-1 Commonly Prescribed Medications (Continued)

TABLE **4-1** Commonly Prescribed Medications (*Continued*)

Name	Classification	Major Therapeutic Uses
clonazepam	benzodiazepine (sedative/ hypnotic, anticonvulsant, anxiolytic)	epilepsy, seizures, anxiety (panic disorder)
clonidine	α_2-adrenergic agonist (antihypertensive)	hypertension
Combivent (ipratropium and albuterol) inhalation aerosol	anticholinergic and adrenergic agonist combination (bronchodilators)	asthma, chronic bronchitis, emphysema
Concerta (methylphenidate) extended release	CNS stimulant	ADHD
Coreg (carvedilol)	cardioselective β-blocker (antihypertensive, antiarrhythmic, antianginal)	hypertension, CHF

Name	Classification	Major Therapeutic Uses
Coumadin (warfarin sodium)	anticoagulant	thromboembolic disorders
Cozaar (losartan)	angiotensin-receptor blocker (antihypertensive)	hypertension
Crestor (rosuvastatin)	HMG-CoA reductase inhibitor (statin)	hyperlipidemia, hypercholesterolemia
Cymbalta (duloxetine hydrochloride)	SSNRI	major depression, diabetic peripheral neuropathic pain
Depakote (divalproex)	anticonvulsant	epilepsy, migraine prophylaxis, bipolar mania
Detrol LA (tolterodine)	anticholinergic	overactive bladder
diazepam	benzodiazepine (sedative/hypnotic, anticonvulsant, anxiolytic)	anxiety, skeletal muscle spasm, epilepsy, seizures

TABLE 4-1 Commonly Prescribed Medications (Continued)

TABLE 4-1	Commonly Prescribed Medications *(Continued)*	
Name	**Classification**	**Major Therapeutic Uses**
Digitek (digoxin)	cardiac glycoside	CHF, cardiac tachyarrhythmias
digoxin	cardiac glycoside	CHF, cardiac tachyarrhythmias
Dilantin (phenytoin)	hydantoin (anticonvulsant)	epilepsy, seizures
Diovan (valsartan)	angiotensin-receptor blocker (antihypertensive)	hypertension
Ditropan XL (oxybutynin)	anticholinergic (urinary antispasmodic)	overactive bladder
doxycycline	tetracycline (antibiotic)	bacterial, rickettsial, chlamydial infections
Effexor XR (venlafaxine)	antidepressant	depression

TABLE 4-1	Commonly Prescribed Medications (*Continued*)	
Name	Classification	Major Therapeutic Uses
Endocet (oxycodone and acetaminophen)	opiate (narcotic) and NSAID (analgesic/antipyretic) combination	moderate to severe pain
estradiol	estrogen	contraception, menstrual irregularity, hormone replacement, vaginal atrophy
Evista (raloxifene)	SERM	prevention and treatment of osteoporosis
famotidine	Antiulcer agent; histamine H_2 agonist	PUD, GERD
fexofenadine	antihistamine	allergy
Flexeril (cyclobenzaprine)	skeletal muscle relaxant	skeletal muscle spasms and spasticity

TABLE 4-1	Commonly Prescribed Medications (Continued)	
Name	**Classification**	**Major Therapeutic Uses**
Flomax (tamsulosin)	α_1-adrenergic antagonist (antihypertensive, vasodilator)	BPH
Flonase (fluticasone) nasal spray	glucocorticoid (anti-inflammatory, immunosuppressant)	allergic rhinitis
Flovent (fluticasone) oral inhalation	glucocorticoid (anti-inflammatory, immunosuppressant)	asthma control
Fosamax (alendronate)	bisphosphonate (bone resorption inhibitor)	osteoporosis, Paget disease
furosemide	diuretic	hypertension, edema associated with CHF or renal disease
gemfibrozil	antihyperlipidemic	hypertriglyceridemia, hyperlipidemia

TABLE 4-1 Commonly Prescribed Medications (*Continued*)

Name	Classification	Major Therapeutic Uses
hydrochlorothiazide	diuretic	hypertension, edema associated with CHF or renal disease
hydrocodone and acetaminophen	opiate (narcotic) and NSAID (analgesic/antipyretic) combination	moderate to severe pain
ibuprofen	analgesic; NSAID	pain, inflammation, fever
Imitrex (sumatriptan succinate)	triptan (antimigraine agent)	migraine headache
Klor-Con (potassium chloride)	potassium salt; electrolyte supplement	potassium deficiency
Lanoxin (digoxin)	cardiac glycoside	CHF, cardiac tachyarrhythmias

4
Med

TABLE 4-1 Commonly Prescribed Medications *(Continued)*

Name	Classification	Major Therapeutic Uses
Levaquin (levofloxacin)	fluoroquinolone (antibiotic)	bacterial infections
Levitra (vardenafil)	phosphodiesterase (type 5) enzyme inhibitor	ED
levothyroxine	thyroid hormone	hypothyroidism
Lexapro (escitalopram)	SSRI (antidepressant)	depression
Lidoderm (lidocaine) patch	local anesthetic	postherpetic neuralgia
Lipitor (atorvastatin)	HMG-CoA reductase inhibitor (statin)	hyperlipidemia, hypercholesterolemia
lithium	disorder	antimanic manic episodes of bipolar

Name	Classification	Major Therapeutic Uses
lorazepam	benzodiazepine (sedative/hypnotic, anticonvulsant, anxiolytic)	anxiety, preoperative sedation, epilepsy, seizures
lovastatin	HMG-CoA reductase inhibitor (statin)	hyperlipidemia, hypercholesterolemia
Lunesta (eszopiclone)	hypnotic	insomnia
Macrobid (nitrofurantoin)	antibiotic	bacterial infections of urinary tract
methylprednisolone	glucocorticoid (anti-inflammatory, immunosuppressant)	inflammation, immunological disorders, allergies
metoclopramide	prokinetic; antiemetic	GERD, gastroparesis, nausea, vomiting

TABLE **4-1** Commonly Prescribed Medications (*Continued*)

TABLE 4-1	Commonly Prescribed Medications (*Continued*)	
Name	Classification	Major Therapeutic Uses
metronidazole	antibacterial, antiprotozoal	bacterial infections, protozoal infections
minocycline	antibiotic	bacterial infections
naproxen	NSAID	pain, inflammation, fever
Nasacort (triamcinolone)	glucocorticoid (anti-inflammatory, immunosuppressant)	allergic rhinitis
Nasonex (mometasone)	glucocorticoid (anti-inflammatory, immunosuppressant)	allergic rhinitis
Nexium (esomeprazole)	PPI (gastric acid secretion inhibitor)	PUD, GERD
nifedipine	calcium-channel blocker	hypertension, angina pectoris

TABLE 4-1 Commonly Prescribed Medications *(Continued)*

Name	Classification	Major Therapeutic Uses
NitroQuick (nitroglycerin)	antianginal	coronary vasodilator
Norvasc (amlodipine)	calcium-channel blocker	hypertension, angina pectoris
nystatin	antifungal	fungus
Omnicef (cefdinir)	cephalosporin (antibiotic)	bacterial infections
OxyContin (oxycodone)	opiate (narcotic) analgesic	moderate to severe pain
Paxil (paroxetinel)	SSRI (antidepressant)	depression
Penicillin VK (penicillin v potassium)	penicillin (antibiotic)	bacterial infections
phenobarbital	barbiturate (sedative/hypnotic, anticonvulsant, anxiolytic)	insomnia, epilepsy, seizures, anxiety
Plavix (clopidogrel)	antiplatelet agent	reduction in stroke or myocardial infarction risk by excessive clot prevention

TABLE 4-1	Commonly Prescribed Medications (*Continued*)	
Name	Classification	Major Therapeutic Uses
Pravachol (pravastatin)	HMG-CoA reductase inhibitor (statin)	hyperlipidemia, hypercholesterolemia
prednisone	glucocorticoid (anti-inflammatory, immunosuppressant)	inflammation, immunological disorders, allergy
Premarin (conjugated estrogens)	estrogen derivative	hormone replacement
Prempro (estrogen and medroxyprogesterone)	estrogen/progestin	hormone replacement
Prevacid (lansoprazole)	PPI (gastric acid secretion inhibitor)	PUD, GERD
Prilosec (omeprazole)	PPI (gastric acid secretion inhibitor)	PUD, GERD

TABLE 4-1 Commonly Prescribed Medications (*Continued*)

Name	Classification	Major Therapeutic Uses
Proscar (finasteride)	5α-reductase inhibitor	BPH
Protonix (pantoprazole)	PPI (gastric acid secretion inhibitor)	PUD, GERD
Pulmicort (budesonide) inhalant	glucocorticoid (anti-inflammatory, immunosuppressant)	asthma
ranitidine	H₂ receptor antagonist	PUD, GERD
Rhinocort Aqua (budesonide)	glucocorticoid (anti-inflammatory, immunosuppressant)	allergic rhinitis
Singulair (montelukast)	leukotriene-receptor antagonist	asthma
Skelaxin (metaxalone)	skeletal muscle relaxant	skeletal muscle spasms and spasticity
Spiriva (tiotropium bromide) inhaler	anticholinergic	bronchospasm, as seen in bronchitis, emphysema or COPD

TABLE **4-1** Commonly Prescribed Medications (*Continued*)

Name	Classification	Major Therapeutic Uses
Strattera (atomoxetine)	SNRI	ADHD
Synthroid (levothyroxine)	thyroid product	hypothyroidism
Tamiflu (oseltamivir)	antiviral	viral infections
tetracycline	antibiotic	
Topamax (topiramate)	anticonvulsant	epilepsy (partial seizures)
Toprol-XL (metoprolol)	cardioselective β-blocker (antihypertensive, antiarrhythmic, antianginal)	hypertension, angina pectoris, CHF
tramadol	opioid analgesic	chronic pain
Trimox (amoxicillin)	penicillin (antibiotic)	bacterial infections
Tussionex (hydrocodone and chlorpheniramine)	narcotic antitussive and antihistamine combination	cough and cold

TABLE 4-1	Commonly Prescribed Medications (*Continued*)	
Name	Classification	Major Therapeutic Uses
Valtrex (valacyclovir)	antiviral	herpes viruses
verapamil	calcium-channel blocker	hypertension, cardiac arrhythmias, angina pectoris
Viagra (sildenafil)	phosphodiesterase (type 5) enzyme inhibitor	ED
Vytorin (ezetimibe and simvastatin)	cholesterol absorption inhibitor and HMG-CoA reductase inhibitor (statin) combination	hyperlipidemia, hypercholesterolemia
warfarin	anticoagulant	thromboembolic disorders
Wellbutrin SR (bupropion)	atypical antidepressant	depression
Yasmin 28 (drospirenone and ethinyl estradiol)	oral contraceptive	birth control
Zetia (ezetimibe)	cholesterol absorption inhibitor	hypercholesterolemia

TABLE 4-1 Commonly Prescribed Medications (Continued)

Name	Classification	Major Therapeutic Uses
Zithromax (azithromycin dihydrate)	macrolide (antibiotic)	bacterial infections
Zocor (simvastatin)	HMG-CoA reductase inhibitor (statin)	hyperlipidemia, hypercholesterolemia
Zoloft (sertraline)	selective serotonin reuptake inhibitor (SSRI) (antidepressant)	depression
Zyprexa (olanzapine)	atypical antipsychotic (neuroleptic)	psychoses (e.g., schizophrenia)
Zyrtec (cetirizine)	antihistamine	allergy

ACE, angiotensin-converting enzyme; ADHD, attention-deficit/hyperactivity disorder; BPH, benign prostatic hyperplasia; CNS, central nervous system; COPD, chronic obstructive pulmonary disease; CHF, congestive heart failure; DM, diabetes mellitus; ED, erectile dysfunction; GERD, gastroesophageal reflux disease; NSAID, nonsteroidal anti-inflammatory drug; PUD, peptic ulcer disease; PPI, proton-pump inhibitor; SERM, selective estrogen-receptor modulator; SNRI, selective norepinephrine reuptake inhibitor; SSNRI, selective serotonin and norepinephrine reuptake inhibitor.
From RxList Top 300 Drugs of 2005, available online at www.rxlist.com/top200.htm, and *Stedman's Medical Dictionary for the Health Professions and Nursing*, 5th ed. Baltimore: Lippincott Williams & Wilkins, Appendix listing of *Commonly Prescribed Drugs and Their Applications*.

TABLE **4-2**	Approximate Equivalents (Metric, Apothecary, Household)	
Metric	Apothecary	Household
60 mg	gr i	
0.06 mL	minim i	1 drop
1.0 g	gr xv	
1.0 mL	minim xv	$^1/_5$ tsp
5.0 mL	1 dram	1 tsp
15 mL	$^1/_2$ oz	1 Tbsp
30 mL	1 oz	2 Tbsp
500 mL	16 oz	1 pint
1000 mL	32 oz	1 quart

Reprinted with permission from Taylor C, Lillis C, Le Mone P. *Fundamentals of Nursing: The Art and Science of Nursing Care,* 2nd ed. Philadelphia: Lippincott Williams & Wilkins, 1993;1347.

BOX 4-2 Seven Rights of Medication Administration

1. Right patient
2. Right time and frequency
3. Right dose
4. Right route of administration
5. Right drug
6. Right technique
7. Right documentation

BOX 4-3 Dosage Calculation Formulas

- Ratio/proportion:
- Dose on hand (DH): known quantity (KQ) = dose desired (DD): unknown quantity (UQ)
- Multiply the extremes (DH × UQ). Multiply the means (KQ × DD). Divide the product of the means by the product of the extremes to arrive at the dosage.
- Formula:

$$\frac{\text{Dosage desired}}{\text{Dosage desired}} \times \text{quantity} \times \left(\frac{DD}{DH} \times Q = X \right)$$

- Body surface area:

$$\frac{\text{BSA in } m^2 \times \text{adult dose}}{1.7} = \text{child's dose}$$

BOX 4-3 **Dosage Calculation Formulas** *(Cont.)*

Nomogram for Estimating the Surface Area
of Older Children and Adults

Height		Surface Area	Weight	
feet	centimeters	in square meters	pounds	kilograms

To determine the surface area of the patient, draw a straight line between the point representing the height on the left verticle scale and the point representing the weight on the right vertical scale. The point at which this line intersects the middle verticle scale represents the patient's surface area in square meters. (Used with permission of Ross Products Division, Abbott Laboratories, Inc., Columbus, Ohio.)

Procedure 4-1 Preparing Injections

Equipment
- Physician's order
- Medication for injection
- Antiseptic wipes
- Needle and syringe
- Small gauze pad
- Patient's medical record

1. Review the medication order.
2. Select the medication.
3. Compare the label to the physician's instructions.
4. Check the expiration date.
5. Check the label three times.
6. Calculate the dosage.
7. Choose the needle and syringe.
8. Open the needle and syringe package. Assemble if necessary. Attach needle firmly to the syringe.
9. Withdraw the medication:
   (a) *From an ampule:*
      (1) Tap the ampule stem lightly with fingertips, wrap a piece of gauze around the ampule neck, grasp firmly and snap the stem off. Place ampule top in a sharps container.
      (2) Remove the needle guard and insert the needle lumen below the level of the medication. Withdraw the medication and dispose of ampule in a sharps container.
      (3) Remove any air bubbles. Draw back on the plunger then push it forward to eject the air.
   (b) *From a vial:*
      (1) Cleanse the vial's rubber stopper.
      (2) Remove the needle guard and pull back on the plunger to fill the syringe with an amount of air equal to the amount of medication to be removed from the vial.

(3) Insert the needle into the vial and inject air from the syringe into the vial.
(4) Invert the vial and withdraw medication into the syringe.
(5) Displace any air bubbles in the syringe.
(6) Push the plunger slowly and force the air into the vial.
10. Recap the needle.

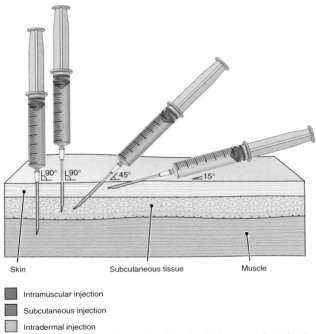

Figure 4-1. Comparison of the angles of insertion for intramuscular, subcutaneous, and intradermal injections. (From Cohen BJ. *Medical Terminology: An Illustrated Guide.* Philadelphia: Lippincott Williams & Wilkins, 2003.)

Procedure 4-2 Intradermal Injection

Equipment
- Physician's order
- Medication for injection
- Antiseptic wipes
- Needle and syringe
- Small gauze pad
- Patient's medical record

 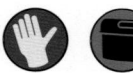

1. Review the medication order.
2. Select the medication.
3. Compare the label to the physician's instructions.
4. Check the expiration date.
5. Check the label three times.
6. Prepare the injection (see Procedure 4-1).
7. Check for medication allergies.
8. Select injection site.
9. Cleanse the site.
10. Put on gloves.
11. Remove needle guard and pull the patient's skin taut.
12. Insert needle at a 10- to 15-degree angle (see Fig. 4-1).
13. Inject the medication. Note that a wheal will form.
14. Remove the needle and dispose of it in sharps container; do not recap.
15. Remove gloves and wash your hands.
16. Perform one of the following tasks at the appropriate time depending on the purpose of the intradermal injection:
    (a) Read the test results. Inspect and palpate the site for the presence and amount of induration.
    (b) Tell the patient when to return (date and time) to the office to have the results read.
    (c) Instruct the patient to read the results at home.
17. Document the procedure.

05/04/08 **10:35 AM**	Mantoux test, 0.1 mL PPD ID, (L) anterior forearm. Pt. given verbal and written instructions to RTO in 48–72 hrs to have results read. Pt. verbalized understanding.
	———————— P. King, CMA

WARNING ⚠️

When removing the needle:
- Do not use an antiseptic wipe or gauze pad.
- Do not press or massage the site.
- Do not apply an adhesive bandage.

Procedure 4-3 Subcutaneous Injection

Equipment
- Physician's order
- Medication for injection
- Antiseptic wipes
- Needle and syringe
- Small gauze pad
- Adhesive bandage
- Patient's medical record

1. Review the medication order.
2. Select the medication.
3. Compare the label to the physician's instructions.
4. Check the expiration date.

5. Check the label three times.
6. Prepare the injection (see Procedure 4-1).
7. Check for medication allergies.
8. Select injection site.
9. Cleanse the site.
10. Put on gloves.
11. Remove the needle guard and hold the injection site in a cushion fashion.
12. Insert the needle at a 45-degree angle (see Fig. 4-1).
13. Remove your nondominant hand from the skin.
14. Pull back on the syringe and inject the medication slowly.
15. Place a gauze pad over the injection site and remove the needle; do not recap.
16. Massage injection site while discarding needle and syringe in sharps container.
17. Apply adhesive bandage if needed.
18. Remove gloves and wash your hands.
19. Alert the physician if any unusual reactions occur.
20. Document the procedure.

CHARTING EXAMPLE

03/04/08 9:30 AM	Regular insulin 5 units SQ (R) posterior upper arm.
	—————————— M. Collins, CMA

Procedure 4-4   Intramuscular Injection

Equipment
- Physician's order
- Medication for injection
- Antiseptic wipes
- Needle and syringe
- Small gauze pad
- Adhesive bandage
- Patient's medical record

1. Review the medication order.
2. Select the correct medication.
3. Compare the label to the physician's instructions.
4. Check the expiration date.
5. Check the label three times.
6. Prepare the injection (see Procedure 4-1).
7. Check for medication allergies.
8. Select injection site (Figs. 4-2 to 4-6).
9. Cleanse the site.
10. Put on gloves.
11. Remove the needle guard. Hold the skin taut in average adult; bunch the muscle in a very thin person.
12. Insert the needle at a 90-degree angle to the hub (see Fig. 4-1).
13. Pull back on the plunger and inject medication.
14. Place a gauze pad over the injection site and remove needle; do not recap.
15. Massage injection site while discarding the needle and syringe in sharps container.
16. Apply adhesive bandage if needed.
17. Remove gloves and wash your hands.
18. Alert the physician if any unusual reactions occur.
19. Document the procedure.

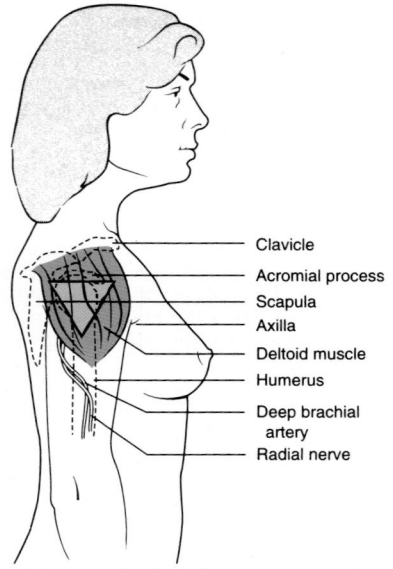

Clavicle

Acromial process

Scapula

Axilla

Deltoid muscle

Humerus

Deep brachial
  artery

Radial nerve

Figure 4-2. The deltoid muscle site for intramuscular injections is located by palpating the lower edge of the acromial process. At the midpoint, in line with the axilla on the lateral aspect of the upper arm, a triangle is formed.

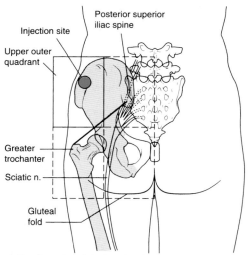

Figure 4-3. The dorsogluteal site for administering an intramuscular injection is lateral and slightly superior to the midpoint of a line drawn from the trochanter to the posterior superior iliac spine. Correct identification of this site minimizes the possibility of accidentally damaging the sciatic nerve.

Labels in figure:
- Posterior superior iliac spine
- Injection site
- Upper outer quadrant
- Greater trochanter
- Sciatic n.
- Gluteal fold

CHARTING EXAMPLE

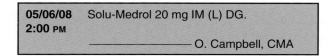

05/06/08 2:00 PM	Solu-Medrol 20 mg IM (L) DG.
	———————— O. Campbell, CMA

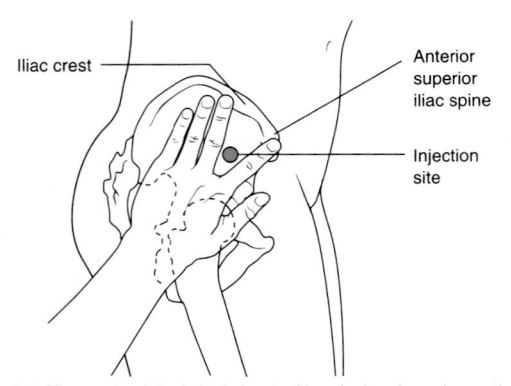

Iliac crest

Anterior
superior
iliac spine

Injection
site

Figure 4-4. The ventrogluteal site is located by placing the palm on the greater trochanter and the index finger toward the anterior superior iliac spine. The middle finger is then spread posteriorly away from the index finger as far as possible. A "V" triangle is formed by this maneuver. The injection is made in the middle of the triangle.

Procedure 4-5   Intramuscular Injection Using the Z-Track Method

Equipment
- Physician's order
- Medication for injection
- Antiseptic wipes
- Needle and syringe
- Small gauze pad
- Adhesive bandage
- Patient's medical record

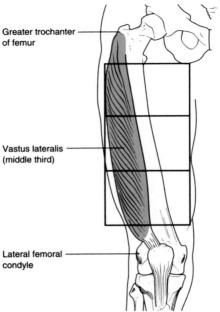

Greater trochanter
of femur

Vastus lateralis
(middle third)

Lateral femoral
condyle

Figure 4-5. The vastus lateralis site for intramuscular injections is identified by dividing the thigh into thirds horizontally and vertically. The injection is given in the outer middle third.

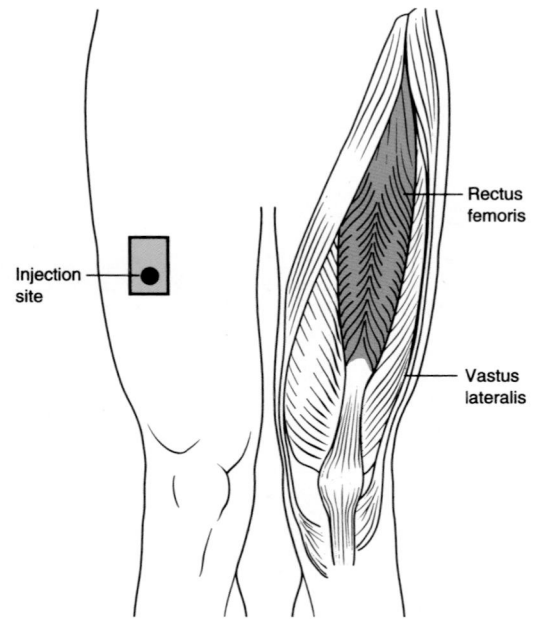

Figure 4-6. The rectus femoris site for intramuscular injections is used only when other sites are contraindicated.

1. Follow steps 1 to 10 in Procedure 4-4: Intramuscular Injection. Note: The ventrogluteal, vastus lateralis, and dorsogluteal sites work well for the Z-track method; the deltoid does not.
2. Remove the needle guard.
3. Pull the top layer of skin to one side with the edge of your nondominant hand.
4. Use a quick, firm motion to insert the needle at a 90-degree angle to the skin.
5. Keep holding the skin to one side with the nondominant hand.
6. Aspirate by withdrawing the plunger slightly, then push the plunger in slowly and steadily. Count to 10 before with-drawing needle.
7. Remove needle while releasing the skin. Do not massage the area.
8. Discard needle and syringe in sharps container; do not recap.
9. Apply adhesive bandage if needed.
10. Remove gloves and wash your hands.
11. Alert the physician if any unusual reactions occur.
12. Document the procedure.

CHARTING EXAMPLE

07/11/08 3:30 PM	Imferon 25mg IM Z-track (R) DG.
	——————————— E. Edwards, CMA

WARNING ⚠

When administering subcutaneous or IM injections:
- Check if blood appears in the hub or syringe (a blood vessel has been entered).
- Do not inject the medication.
- Remove the needle and prepare a new injection.

Procedure 4-6 Applying Transdermal Medications

Equipment
- Physician's order
- Medication
- Patient's medical record

1. Review the medication order.
2. Select the correct medication.
3. Compare the label to the physician's instructions.
4. Check the expiration date.
5. Check the label three times.
6. Check for medication allergies.
7. Select the site and perform skin preparation.
8. If a transdermal patch is already in place:
   (a) Put on gloves and remove patch; discard.
   (b) Inspect the site for irritation.
9. Open the medication package.
10. Apply the patch.
11. Wash your hands.
12. Document the procedure.

Procedure 4-7 Obtaining and Preparing an Intravenous Site

Equipment
- Physician's order including the type of fluid to be used and the rate
- Intravenous solution
- Infusion administration set
- IV pole
- Blank labels
- IV catheter (Angiocath)
- Antiseptic wipes
- Tourniquet
- Small gauze pad
- Bandage tape
- Adhesive bandage
- Patient medical record

1. Review the physician's order.
2. Select the correct catheter, solution, and administration set.
3. Compare the solution label to the physician's order.
4. Note expiration dates for solution and administration set.
5. Label the solution with date, time, and patient's name.
6. Hang the solution on an IV pole.
7. Remove administration set from the package and close the roller clamp.
8. Remove the end of the administration set by removing the spike cover.
9. Remove the cover from the infusion port and insert the spike end of the administration set into the IV fluid.
10. Fill the drip chamber about half full.
11. Open the roller clamp and allow fluid to flow from the drip chamber through the length of the tubing, displacing any air. Do not remove the cover protecting the end of the tubing.

12. Close the roller clamp when fluid has filled the tubing and no air is noted.
13. Drape the filled tubing over the IV pole and perform a venipuncture.
14. Check for medication allergies.
15. Prepare the IV start equipment; tear 2 to 3 strips of tape to secure the IV catheter after insertion.
16. Inspect each arm for the best available vein.
17. Put on gloves and apply the tourniquet.
18. Select a vein.
19. Release the tourniquet after palpating if it has been left on for more than 1 minute.
20. Cleanse the site.
21. Anchor the vein to be punctured.
22. Remove the needle cover from the IV catheter.
23. Insert the needle and catheter unit directly into the top of the vein. Keep the needle bevel up at a 15- to 20-degree angle for superficial veins. Hold the catheter by the flash chamber, not the needle hub. Watch for blood in the flash chamber.
24. Lower the needle angle until flush with the skin; advance the needle and catheter unit about $\frac{1}{4}$ inch and stop.
25. Hold the flash chamber steady with nondominant hand and slide the catheter off the needle and into the vein with dominant hand. The catheter should be advanced into the vein up to the hub.
26. Release the tourniquet.
27. Remove needle and discard in sharps container.
28. Connect the end of the administration tubing to the end of the IV catheter that has been inserted into the vein. Open the roller clamp and adjust the flow.
29. Tape the IV catheter in place.
30. Apply adhesive dressing over the hub and insertion site.
31. Make a small loop with the administration set tubing near the IV insertion site; tape securely.
32. Remove gloves and wash your hands.
33. Document the procedure.

Procedure 4-8 Instilling Eye Medications

Equipment
- Physician's order
- Patient record
- Ophthalmic medication
- Sterile gauze
- Tissues

1. Obtain the patient's medical record, physician's order, correct medication, sterile gauze, and tissues.
2. Check the label three times.
3. Check for medication allergies.
4. Position the patient comfortably.
5. Put on gloves.
6. Pull down the lower eyelid with sterile gauze and have the patient look up.
7. Instill the medication:

   Ointment
   - Discard the first bead of ointment onto a tissue.
   - Place a thin line of ointment across the inside of the lower eyelid.
   - Twist the tube to release the ointment.
   - Do not touch the tube to the eye.

   Drops
   - Hold the dropper close to the conjunctival sac.
   - Release the proper number of drops into the sac.
   - Discard any medication left in the dropper.
8. Release the lower lid and have the patient close the eye and roll it to disperse the medication.
9. Tissue off any excess medication.
10. Have the patient apply light pressure to the puncta lacrimalis for several minutes.
11. Care for or dispose of equipment.

12. Clean the work area and wash your hands.
13. Record the procedure.

Procedure 4-9 Instilling Ear Medications

Equipment
- Physician's order
- Patient's record
- Otic medication with dropper
- Cotton balls

1. Check the medication label three times.
2. Seat the patient with affected ear tilted upward.
3. Draw up the ordered medication amount.
4. Straighten the ear canal.
   - *Adults:* Pull the auricle slightly up and back.
   - *Children:* Pull the auricle slightly down and back.
5. Insert the dropper tip without touching the ear and let the medication flow.
6. Have the patient sit or lie with the affected ear up for about 5 minutes.
7. If medication is to be retained in the ear canal, insert a moist cotton ball into the external auditory meatus.
8. Care for or dispose of equipment.
9. Clean the work area and wash your hands.
10. Record the procedure

Procedure 4-10 Instilling Nasal Medications

Equipment
- Physician's order
- Patient's record

- Nasal medication
- Drops or spray
- Tissues

1. Check the medication label three times.
2. Check for medication allergies.
3. Position the patient recumbent, head tilted back.
4. Administer the medication.
   (a) Hold dropper upright and dispense one drop at a time. Have patient remain recumbent for 5 minutes.
   (b) Place the tip of the bottle at the naris opening and spray as the patient takes a deep breath.
5. Tissue off excess medication.
6. Care for or dispose of equipment. Clean the work area.
7. Remove gloves and wash your hands.
8. Record the procedure.

Procedure 4-11 Nebulized Breathing Treatment

Equipment
- Physician order
- Patient's medical record
- Inhalation medication
- Saline for inhalation
- Nebulizer disposable setup
- Nebulizer

1. Check the medication label three times.
2. Add medication to the nebulizer treatment cup.

3. Add 2 to 3 mL saline for inhalation therapy to the cup. (Many nebulizer medications are pre-packaged with saline. It may not be necessary to add additional saline if this is the case).
4. Place the top on the cup, attach the T piece to the top of the cup, and position the mouthpiece firmly on one end of the T piece.
5. Attach one end of the tubing to the connector on the cup and the other end to the connector on the nebulizer machine.
6. Instruct the patient to put in the mouthpiece and breathe normally during treatment.
7. Turn the machine on. The medication in the cup becomes a fine mist for the patient to inhale.
8. Record the patient's pulse before, during, and after treatment.
9. Turn off the machine and have the patient remove the mouthpiece.
10. Disconnect the disposable treatment setup.
11. Dispose of all parts in a biohazard container and put away the machine.
12. Wash your hands and document the procedure.

CHARTING EXAMPLE

11/26/08 **9:15 AM**	Pt. given nebulized breathing treatment with Ipratropium Bromide 0.5 mg and albuterol sulfate 3.0 mg for inhalation – pulse before treatment 88, during treatment 100, and after treatment 110. Pt. states she is "breathing easier" after treatment, skin warm and dry, color pink.

———————————— J. Baker, CMA

5 Surgical Procedures

BOX 5-1 **Maintaining Sterility**

Follow these guidelines to maintain sterility before and during a sterile procedure:
1. Do not let sterile packages get damp or wet.
2. Always face a sterile field.
3. Hold all sterile items above waist level.
4. Presume that sterile items not in your field of vision have become contaminated.
5. Place sterile items in the middle of the sterile field.
6. Do not spill *any* liquids onto the sterile field.
7. Do not cough, sneeze, or talk over the sterile field.
8. Never reach over the sterile field.
9. Do not pass soiled supplies over the sterile field.

Procedure 5-1 Opening Sterile Surgical Packs

Equipment
- Surgical pack
- Surgical or Mayo stand
- Additional sterile drape

1. Verify the procedure to be performed.
2. Obtain the surgical package.
3. Check the contents and expiration date.
4. Check for tears and moisture.
5. Place the package, label up, on Mayo or surgical stand.
6. Remove the sealing tape. With commercial packages, remove the outer protective wrapper.
7. Open the first flap away from you.
8. Open the side flaps.
9. Pull the remaining flap down and toward you.
10. Repeat steps 7 to 9 for packages with a second or inside wrapper.
11. Cover with a sterile drape if you must leave after opening the field.

WARNING

If you suspect the field has been contaminated, view the field as nonsterile. Begin the procedure again with new, sterile supplies and equipment.

Procedure 5-2   Using Sterile Transfer Forceps

Equipment
- Sterile transfer forceps in a container with sterilization solution
- Sterile field
- Sterile items to be transferred

1. Lift the forceps out of the container.
2. Hold the forceps with tips down and above waist level.
3. Pick up items to be transferred and drop them onto the sterile field. Do not let the forceps touch the sterile field.
4. Place the forceps back in the sterilization solution.

Procedure 5-3   Adding Sterile Solution to a Sterile Field

Equipment
- Sterile setup
- Container of sterile solution
- Sterile bowl or cup

1. Identify the correct solution.
2. Check the expiration date.
3. If you are adding medication, show the label to the physician.
4. Remove cap or stopper. Hold the cap facing downward.
5. Grasp container with the label against your palm.
6. Pour a small amount of solution into a separate container or waste receptacle.
7. Pour the desired amount of solution into the sterile container. Avoid splashing.
8. Recheck the label and expiration date; replace the cap.
9. Store or discard the solution.

Procedure 5-4   Hair Removal and Skin Preparation

Equipment
- Shave cream, lotion, or soap
- New disposable razor
- Gauze or cotton balls
- Warm water
- Antiseptic
- Sponge forceps

1. Put on gloves and prepare skin:
   (a) *Shaving:* Apply shaving cream, pull skin taut, and shave in direction of hair growth. Rinse and pat dry with gauze square.
   (b) *Non-shaving:* Wash and rinse with soap and water; dry.
2. Apply antiseptic solution to skin surrounding the operative area.
3. Wipe the skin in circular motions.
4. Discard each gauze or cotton ball after a complete sweep.
5. Hold dry sterile gauze sponges in the sponge forceps and pat area dry.
6. Instruct the patient not to touch or cover the prepared area.
7. Inform physician that the patient is ready.

Procedure 5-5 Applying Sterile Gloves

Equipment
   • Package of sterile gloves

1. Remove rings and other jewelry.
2. Wash hands.
3. Place packaged gloves on clean, dry, flat surface, cuffed end toward you.
4. Pull outer wrapping apart to expose sterile inner wrap (Fig. 5-1).
5. Fold back inner wrap to expose gloves (Fig. 5-2).
6. Grasp edges and open the package (Fig. 5-3).

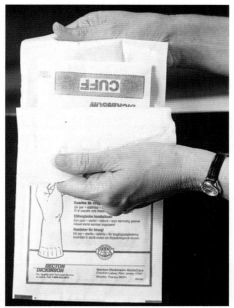

Figure 5-1.

7. Using your nondominant hand, lift the cuff of the glove for the dominant hand, touching only the inner surface. Curl your thumb inward as you insert hand (Fig. 5-4).
8. Curl your fingers and thumb together and insert them into glove. Straighten your fingers and pull the glove on with your nondominant hand while still grasping the cuff.

9. Unfold the cuff; pinch the inside surface that will be against your wrist and pull it toward the wrist.

10. Pull the glove on snugly, touching only the inside surface of the cuff (Fig. 5-5).

11. Place gloved fingers under the cuff of the remaining glove. Lift the glove up and away from the wrapper, and slide in your ungloved hand with your fingers and thumb curled together (Fig. 5-6).

12. Unfold cuff and pull the glove on (Fig. 5-7).

13. Adjust the fingers for a comfortable fit (Fig. 5-8).
    (To remove contaminated sterile gloves, see Procedure 2-2.)

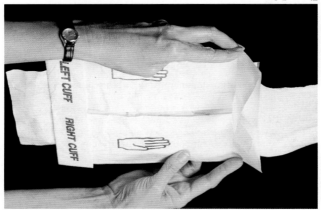

Figure 5-2.

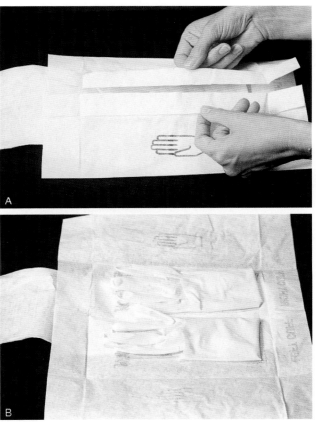

Figure 5-3.

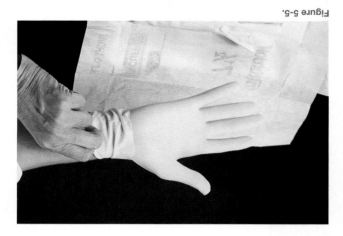

Figure 5-5.

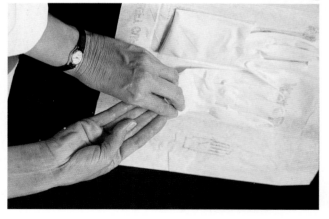

Figure 5-4.

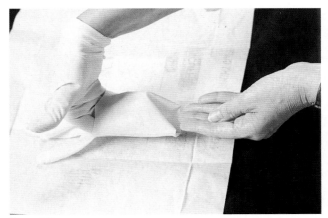

Figure 5-6.

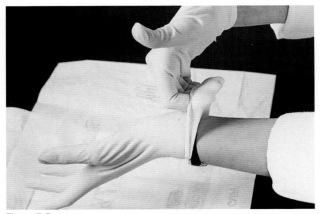

Figure 5-7.

151

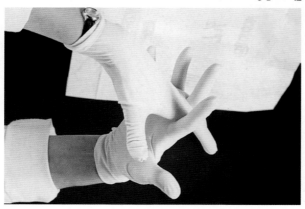

Figure 5-8.

Procedure 5-6 Apply a Sterile Dressing

Equipment
- Sterile gauze dressings
- Scissors
- Bandage tape
- Medication, if ordered

1. Check for tape allergies.
2. Cut lengths of tape to secure the dressing; set aside.
3. Instruct the patient to remain still.
4. Open the dressing pack to create a sterile field.

5. To maintain sterility:
    (a) *If using sterile gloves:* Put on gloves before touching sterile items.
    (b) *If using sterile transfer forceps:* Use sterile technique to arrange dressing on the wound.
6. Apply medication, if ordered.
7. Apply the number of dressings necessary to cover and protect the wound.
8. Secure the dressing with tape.
9. Discard gloves.
10. Provide patient instruction on dressing changes.
11. Wear clean examination gloves to care for or dispose of equipment.
12. Clean the work area, remove gloves, and wash your hands.
13. Return reusable supplies to storage area.
14. Record the procedure.

Procedure 5-7 Changing an Existing Sterile Dressing

Equipment
- Sterile dressing
- Prepackaged skin antiseptic swabs, or sterile antiseptic solution in a sterile basin and sterile cotton balls or gauze
- Tape

1. Prepare a sterile field, including opening sterile dressings and antiseptic solution.
2. Instruct the patient to remain still.
3. Put on clean gloves.
4. Remove dressing tape, then remove the dressing.
5. Discard soiled dressing in biohazard container. Do not pass it over the sterile field.

6. Inspect wound for healing, drainage amount and type, and wound edge appearance.
7. Remove and discard gloves.
8. Put on sterile gloves.
9. Clean the wound with antiseptic solution.
10. Remove gloves and wash your hands.
11. Change the dressing (see Procedure 5-6).
12. Record the procedure.

WARNING ⚠

Never pull on a dressing that does not come off easily; you may disrupt the healing process.

BOX 5-2 **Bandaging Guidelines**

- Observe medical asepsis.
- Keep the wound dressing and bandage dry to avoid wicking microorganisms to the site.
- Never place bandages against a wound: Dressings cover the wound; bandages cover the dressing and should extend at least 1 inch beyond the dressing.
- Do not dress skin surfaces together; pad opposing surfaces to prevent tissues from adhering during healing.
- Pad joints and bony surfaces to prevent friction.
- Bandage a part in its normal, slightly flexed position to avoid muscle strain.
- Begin the bandage distally and work proximally.
- Assess the patient's level of discomfort; adjust the bandage for comfort and security.
- When bandaging extremities, leave the fingers or toes exposed for evaluating circulation.

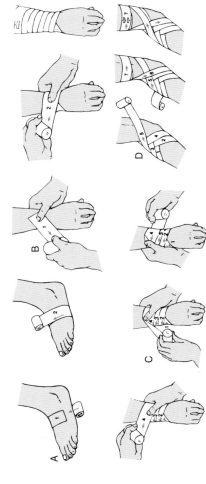

Figure 5-9. There are six basic techniques for wrapping a roller bandage. **(A)** A circular turn is used to anchor and secure a bandage when it is started and ended. It simply involves holding the free end of the rolled material in one hand and wrapping it about the area, bringing it back to the starting point. **(B)** A spiral turn partly overlaps a previous turn. The overlapping varies from one-half to three-fourths the width of the bandage. Spiral turns are used when wrapping a cylindrical part of the body, such as the arm or leg. **(C)** A spiral-reverse turn is a modification of a spiral turn. The roll is reversed halfway through the turn. This works well on tapered body parts. **(D)** A figure-eight turn is best used when an area spanning a joint, such as the elbow or knee, requires bandaging. It is made by making oblique turns that alternately ascend and descend, simulating a figure eight.

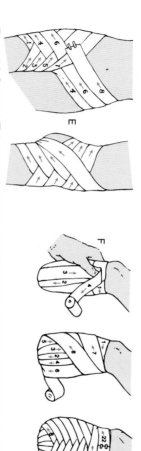

Figure 5-9. *Continued.* **(E)** A spica turn is a variation of the figure-eight turn. It differs in that the wrap includes a portion of the trunk or chest. **(F)** The recurrent turn is made by passing the roll back and forth over the tip of a body part. Once several recurrent turns have been make, the bandage is anchored by completing the application with another basic turn, such as the figure eight. A recurrent turn is especially beneficial when wrapping the stump of an amputated limb.

Procedure 5-8 Assisting with Excisional Surgery

Equipment
- *At the side:* Sterile gloves, local anesthetic, antiseptic wipes, adhesive tape, specimen container with completed laboratory request.
- *On the field:* Basin for solutions, gauze sponges and cotton balls, antiseptic solution, sterile drape, dissecting scissors, disposable scalpel, blade of physician's choice, mosquito forceps, tissue forceps, needle holder, suture and needle of physician's choice.

1. Set up a sterile field on a surgical stand with at-the-side equipment close at hand.
2. Cover the field with a sterile drape until physician arrives.
3. Position the patient appropriately.
4. Put on sterile gloves or use sterile transfer forceps and cleanse the patient's skin (see Procedure 5-4).
5. Remove gloves (if used) and wash hands.
6. As needed, add supplies, assist the physician, and comfort the patient.
7. Collect the specimen in appropriate container, if lesion requires pathology analysis.
8. When procedure is complete, wash hands and dress the wound using sterile technique (see Procedure 5-6).
9. Provide patient instructions on caring for the operative site, dressing changes, postoperative medications, and follow-up visits.
10. Put on gloves and clean the room.
11. Discard used disposables in biohazard containers. Return unused items to storage.
12. Remove gloves and wash your hands.
13. Record the procedure.

Procedure 5-9 Assisting with Incision and Drainage

Equipment
- *At the side:* sterile gloves, local anesthetic, needle and syringe if not placed on sterile field, antiseptic wipes, adhesive tape, sterile dressings, packing gauze, culture tube if the wound may be cultured.
- *On the field:* basin for solutions, gauze sponges and cotton balls, antiseptic solution, sterile drape, syringes and needles for local anesthetic, commercial I & D sterile setup or scalpel, dissecting scissors, hemostats, tissue forceps, sterile 4 × 4 gauze sponges, sterile probe (optional).

The steps for this procedure are similar to those in Procedure 5-8. You are expected to prepare the surgical field and the patient's surgical area per physician's preference. After the procedure, cover the wound to avoid further contamination and to absorb drainage. The exudate is a hazardous body fluid requiring standard precautions. Although a culture and sensitivity may be ordered on the drainage from the infected area, no other specimen is usually collected.

Procedure 5-10 Removing Sutures

Equipment
- Skin antiseptic
- Prepackaged suture removal kit, or thumb forceps
- Suture scissors
- 2 × 2 gauze

1. If dressing is still in place: Put on clean gloves, remove it, and dispose in biohazard container. Remove gloves and wash your hands.

2. Put on clean gloves and cleanse the wound with an antiseptic (Fig. 5-10).
3. Open the suture removal packet using sterile asepsis or set up a field for on-site sterile equipment. Put on sterile gloves.
4. Knots will be tied so that one tail of the knot is very close to the surface of the skin; the other will be closer to the area of suture that is looped over the incision (Fig. 5-11).
   (a) Use thumb forceps to grasp the end of the knot closest to the skin and lift it up.
   (b) Cut the suture below the knot as close to the skin as possible.
   (c) Use thumb forceps to pull the suture out of the skin.

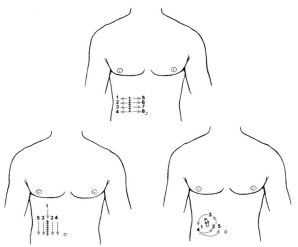

Figure 5-10. Wound cleaning. Clean the wound outward from the site following any of the numbered patterns.

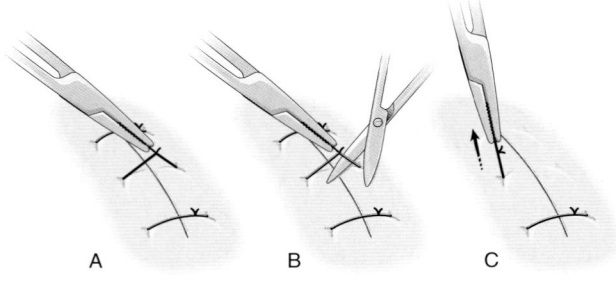

Figure 5-11. (A) With the hemostat or thumb forceps the stitch up and away from the skin. **(B)** Cut stitch near the skin. **(C)** Using the forceps, put freed stitch up and out.

5. Place the suture on the gauze sponge. Repeat the procedure for each suture to be removed.
6. Clean the site with an antiseptic solution, and cover with a sterile dressing if ordered.
7. Care for or dispose of equipment. Clean the work area.
8. Remove gloves and wash your hands.
9. Record the procedure.

CHARTING EXAMPLE

06/26/08	×6 sutures removed from (L) ring finger.
3:30 PM	Wound well approximated, no drainage.
	——————————— J. Rose, RMA

Procedure 5-11 Removing Staples

Equipment
- Antiseptic solution or wipes
- Gauze squares
- Sponge forceps
- Prepackaged sterile staple removal instrument

1. If dressing is still in place: Put on clean gloves, remove it, and dispose in a biohazard container. Remove gloves and wash your hands.
2. Clean the incision with antiseptic solution. Pat dry with sterile gauze sponges.
3. Put on sterile gloves.
4. Slide the end of the staple remover under each staple to be removed. Press the handles together to lift the ends of the staple out of the skin (Fig. 5-12).
5. Place each staple on a gauze square as it is removed.
6. When all staples are removed, clean the incision. Pat dry and dress the site if ordered.
7. Care for or dispose of equipment. Clean the work area.
8. Remove gloves and wash your hands.
9. Record the procedure.

Procedure 5-12 Assisting with Lumbar Puncture

Equipment
- Sterile and clean exam gloves
- 3- to 5- inch lumbar needle with stylet (physician will specify gauge and length)
- Sterile gauze sponges
- Sterile specimen container
- Local anesthetic and syringe

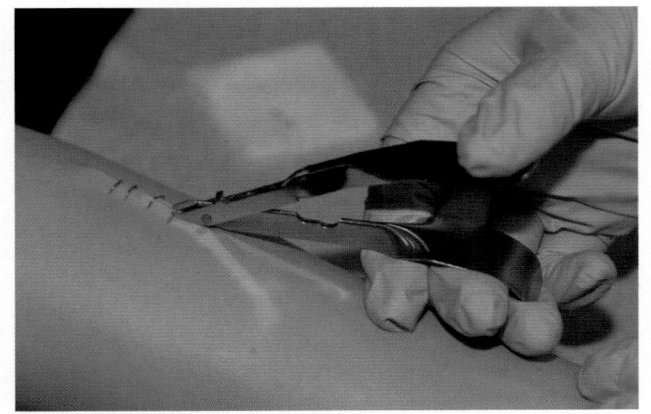

Figure 5-12. Slide the end of the staple remover under each staple. Press the handles together to lift the ends of the staple out of the skin.

- Needle
- Adhesive bandages
- Fenestrated drape
- Sterile drape
- Antiseptic
- Skin preparation supplies (razor)

1. Check that consent form is signed and in the chart.
2. Warn the patient not to move during the procedure.
3. Have the patient void, then disrobe and put on a gown.

4. Prepare the skin (unless this is to be done with sterile preparation).
5. Assist as needed with anesthetic administration.
6. Prepare the sterile field and assist with the initial preparations. Patient positioning:
   • *Side-lying:* Stand in front of the patient and hold the knees and top shoulder.
   • *Forward-leaning:* Stand in front of the patient and rest your hands on the shoulders.
7. During the procedure: Observe for dyspnea or cyanosis. Monitor the pulse and record vital signs after the procedure. Note patient's mental alertness, any leakage at the site, or nausea or vomiting. Assess lower limb mobility.
8. If specimens are to be taken: Put on gloves. Label the tubes in sequence as you receive them. Include patient's identification. Place tubes in biohazard bags.
9. If Queckenstedt test is performed: Press against the patient's jugular veins in the neck (right, left, or both) while the physician monitors the pressure of CSF.
10. When procedure is finished, cover site with an adhesive bandage and assist patient to a flat position.
11. Route specimens.
12. Clean the room. Care for or dispose of the equipment as needed.
13. Wash your hands.
14. Chart observations and record the procedure.

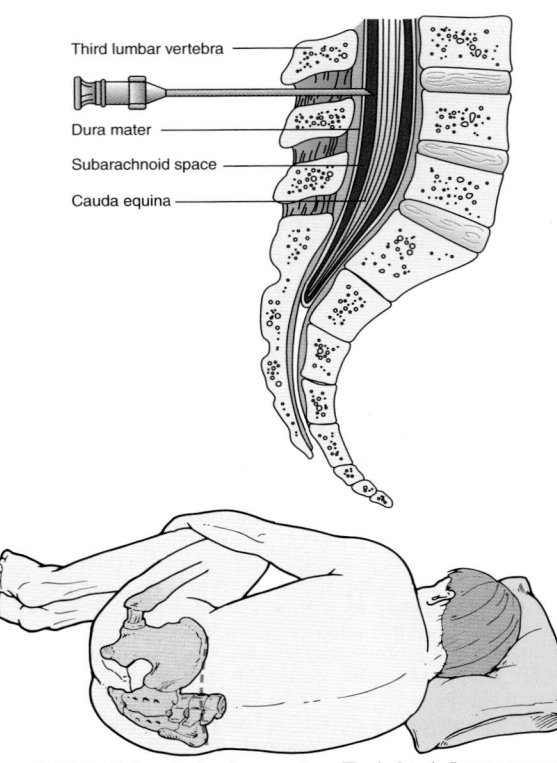

Figure 5-13. Technique for lumbar puncture. The L-3 to L-5 spaces are just below the line connecting the anterior and superior iliac spines. (From Taylor C, Lillis CA, LeMone P. *Fundamentals of Nursing,* 2nd ed. Philadelphia: Lippincott Williams & Wilkins, 1993;543.)

Procedure 5-13 Assisting with Colposcopy and Cervical Biopsy

Equipment
- Gown and drape
- Vaginal speculum
- Colposcope
- Specimen container with preservative (10% formalin)
- Sterile gloves
- Sterile cotton-tipped applicators
- Sterile normal saline solution
- Sterile 3% acetic acid
- Sterile povidone-iodine (Betadine)
- Silver nitrate sticks or ferric subsulfate (Monsel solution)
- Sterile biopsy forceps or punch biopsy instrument
- Sterile uterine curet
- Sterile uterine dressing forceps
- Sterile 4 × 4 gauze
- Sterile towel
- Sterile endocervical curet
- Sterile uterine tenaculum
- Sanitary napkin
- Examination gloves
- Examination light
- Tissues

1. Check that consent form is signed and in chart.
2. Check colposcope light.
3. Set up the sterile field.
4. Pour sterile normal saline and acetic acid into their sterile containers. Cover the field with a sterile drape.
5. Position patient: dorsal lithotomy. If assisting from the sterile field, put on sterile gloves.

165

6. Hand physician the applicator immersed in normal saline, then the applicator immersed in acetic acid.
7. Hand physician the applicator with antiseptic solution (Betadine).
8. If you did not apply sterile gloves, apply clean gloves and receive biopsy specimen into the container of 10% formalin preservative.
9. Give the physician Monsel solution or silver nitrate sticks to stop bleeding if necessary.
10. When procedure is finished, assist patient to a sitting position. Explain that a small amount of bleeding may occur; have a sanitary napkin available.
11. Label specimen container and prepare laboratory request.
12. Provide privacy for dressing.
13. Reinforce physician instructions and tell patient how to obtain the biopsy findings.
14. Care for or dispose of equipment. Clean the room.
15. Wash your hands.
16. Document the procedure.

Special Procedures

6

Procedure 6-1 Applying a Warm or Cold Compress

Equipment
- *Warm compresses:* appropriate solution (water with possible antiseptic if ordered), warmed to 110°F or recommended temperature, bath thermometer, absorbent material (cloth, gauze), waterproof barriers, hot water bottle (optional), clean or sterile basin
- *Cold compresses:* appropriate solution, ice bag or cold pack, absorbent material (cloth, gauze), waterproof barriers

1. Pour solution into the basin. For warm compresses, check the solution's temperature.
2. Have patient remove clothing as appropriate and put on a gown; drape.
3. Protect examination table with a waterproof barrier.
4. Place absorbent material or gauze in the solution. Wring out excess moisture.
5. Lightly place compress on skin and ask the patient about the temperature for comfort.
6. Observe for skin color changes.

167

7. Arrange the compress and contour the material to the area; cover with a waterproof barrier.
8. Check the compress frequently for moisture and temperature. Use hot water bottles or ice packs to maintain temperature; rewet absorbent material as needed.
9. After required time, remove the compress.
10. Discard disposable materials and disinfect reusable equipment.
11. Remove gloves and wash your hands.
12. Document the procedure.

Note: Use sterile technique if applying compress to an area with an open lesion.

Procedure 6-2 Assisting with Therapeutic Soaks

Equipment
- Clean or sterile basin or container in which to place the body part comfortably
- Solution and/or medication
- Dry towels
- Bath thermometer

1. Pad surfaces of container.
2. Fill container with solution and check temperature (should be below 110°F).
3. Slowly lower area to be soaked into container and check patient's reaction.
4. Arrange body part comfortably. Check for pressure areas and pad edges as needed.
5. Check solution temperature every 5 to 10 minutes. If more water or solution must be added to maintain temperature, remove some solution and then add warmed solution,

shielding patient's skin. Mix or swirl to ensure even
temperature.
6. Soak for required time.
7. Remove body part from solution; towel dry.
8. Care for or dispose of equipment.
9. Document the procedure

Procedure 6-3 Applying Cold Packs

Equipment
- Ice bag and ice chips or small cubes, or a disposable cold
  pack
- Small towel or cover for the ice pack
- Gauze or tape

1. If using ice bag, check for leaks. Fill about two-thirds full
   and press flat to express air. Seal bag.
2. If using a chemical ice pack, activate it following manufacturer's instructions.
3. Place cold pack in protective cover.
4. Assess patient's skin for color and warmth, then place
   covered cold pack on the area.
5. Secure cold pack with gauze or tape.
6. Apply treatment for prescribed time, no more than
   30 minutes.
7. Assess skin frequently for mottling, pallor, or redness.
   Remove cold pack immediately if these appear and alert the
   physician.
8. Care for or dispose of equipment. Wash your hands.
9. Document the procedure.

Procedure 6-4 Using a Hot Water Bottle or Commercial Hot Pack

Equipment
- Hot water bottle or commercial hot pack
- Towel or other covering for the hot pack

1. If using a hot water bottle, check for leaks. Fill about two-thirds full with warm (110°F) water; express air before capping.
2. If using a commercial hot pack, activate it following manufacturer's directions.
3. Wrap and secure bottle or pack.
4. Assess skin color, then place covered hot pack on the area. Secure with gauze or tape.
5. Apply treatment for prescribed time, no more than 30 minutes.
6. Assess skin every 10 minutes for pallor, excessive redness, swelling. Remove hot pack immediately if these appear and alert the physician.
7. Care for or dispose of equipment. Wash your hands.
8. Document the procedure.

WARNING

Commercial cold or hot pack activators should be broken gently, as they contain chemicals that can cause burns on contact. Dispose of leaking or broken packs immediately.

TABLE 6-1	Proper Use of Heat and Cold
Do *not use* heat	Within 24 hours after an injury because it may increase bleeding
	For noninflammatory edema because increased capillary permeability allows additional tissue fluid to build up
	In cases of acute inflammation because increased blood supply increases the inflammatory process
	In the presence of malignancies because cell metabolism is enhanced
	Over the pregnant uterus because incidences of genetic mutation have been linked to heat applied to the gravid uterus
	On areas of erythema or vesicles because it compounds the existing problem
	Over metallic implants because it causes discomfort
Do *not use* cold	On open wounds because decreased blood supply delays healing
	In the presence of already-impaired circulation because it further impairs circulation

ORTHOPEDIC PROCEDURES

Procedure 6-5 Applying an Arm Sling

Equipment
  • Canvas arm sling with adjustable straps

1. Position affected limb with the hand at slightly less than a 90-degree angle, fingers slightly higher than elbow.
2. Place elbow into pocket of sling.
3. Bring strap across the back and over the opposite shoulder to the front of the patient.
4. Secure the velcro end of the strap by inserting the end of it under the sling loop.
5. Pull the strap through the loop so the arm and hand remain slightly elevated at 90 degrees.
6. Press the velcro ends together and check the patient's comfort and circulation.
7. Document the appliance in the patient's chart.

CHARTING EXAMPLE

10/28/08 **11:15 AM**	Arm sling applied to (R) arm as ordered. Fingers to (R) hand warm and pink, no swelling. To RTO in 4 days.
	————————— T. Burton, RMA

Procedure 6-6 — Measuring a Patient for Axillary Crutches

Equipment
- Axillary crutches with tips
- Pads for the axilla
- Hand rests as needed

1. Ensure patient is wearing low-heeled shoes with safety soles.
2. Have patient stand erect; provide support as needed.
3. Have patient hold the crutches naturally, in tripod position (tips about 2 inches in front of and 4 to 6 inches to the sides of the feet).
4. Adjust the central support in the base so that axillary bar is about two finger-breadths below the patient's axillae. Tighten bolts for safety.
5. Adjust the handgrips so that the patient's elbow is at a 30-degree angle when gripping the bar. Tighten bolts for safety.
6. If needed, pad axillary bars and handgrips with large gauze pads or small towels; secure with tape.
7. Wash your hands and record the procedure.

Procedure 6-7 — Instructing Patient in Crutch Gaits

1. Have the patient stand up from a chair, holding both crutches on the affected side, then sliding to the edge of the chair.
2. Ensure the patient pushes down on the chair arm on the unaffected side, then pushes to stand. With one crutch in each hand, the patient rests on the crutches until balance is restored.
3. Assist patient to the tripod position.
4. Depending upon weight-bearing ability, coordination, and general state of health, instruct the patient in one or more of the following gaits in Figure 6-1.
5. Wash hands and record the procedure.

173

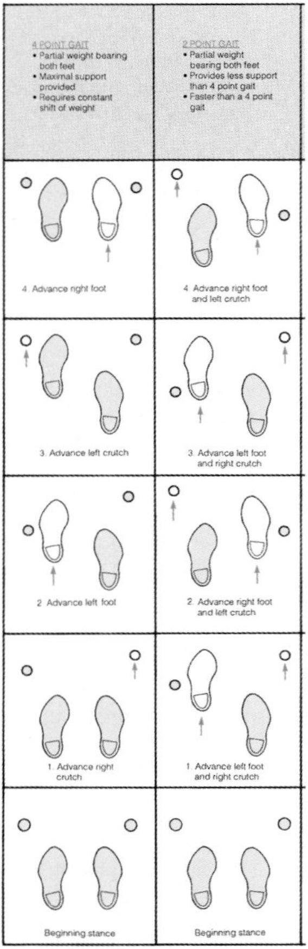

Figure 6-1. Crutch gaits.

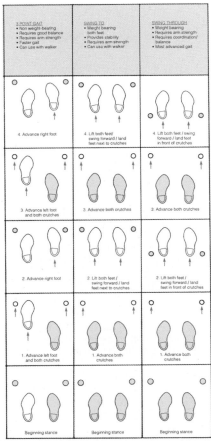

3 POINT GAIT • Non weight-bearing • Requires good balance • Requires arm strength • Faster gait • Can use with walker	SWING TO • Weight bearing both feet • Provides stability • Requires arm strength • Can use with walker	SWING THROUGH • Weight bearing • Requires arm strength • Requires coordination/balance • Most advanced gait
4. Advance right foot	4. Lift both feet/ swing forward / land feet next to crutches	4. Lift both feet / swing forward / land feet in front of crutches
3. Advance left foot and both crutches	3. Advance both crutches	3. Advance both crutches
2. Advance right foot	2. Lift both feet / swing forward / land feet next to crutches	2. Lift both feet / swing forward / land feet in front of crutches
1. Advance left foot and both crutches	1. Advance both crutches	1. Advance both crutches
Beginning stance	Beginning stance	Beginning stance

Figure 6-1. *Continued.*

BOX 6-1   **Climbing and Descending Stairs on Crutches**

Instruct the patient as follows:

Climbing stairs:
* Stand close to the bottom step.
* With weight supported on the hand rests, step up to the first step with the unaffected leg.
* Bring the affected side and crutches up to the step at the same time.
* Resume balance before proceeding to the next step.
* Remember: The good side goes up first!

Descending stairs:
* Stand close to the edge of the top step.
* Bend from the hips and knees to adjust to the height of the lower step. Do not lean forward as this may cause a fall.
* Carefully lower the crutches and affected limb to the next step.
* Next, lower the unaffected leg to the lower step and resume balance. If a handrail is available, hold both crutches in one hand and follow the steps above.
* Remember: The affected foot goes down first!

EYE AND EAR PROCEDURES

Procedure 6-8   Distance Visual Acuity

Equipment
* Snellen eye chart
* Paper cup or eye paddle

1. Escort patient to well-lighted examination area.
2. Ensure chart is at eye level, with a distance marker exactly 20 feet away.
3. Position patient 20 feet from the eye chart.
4. Observe whether the patient is wearing glasses. If not, ask about contact lenses and mark the test results accordingly.
5. Instruct patient to cover left eye and to keep both eyes open during the test.
6. Stand beside the chart and point to each row, starting with the 20/200 line.
7. Record the smallest line that the patient can read with either one or no errors, according to office policy.
8. Repeat the procedure with the right eye covered and record as in step 6.
9. If the patient squints or leans forward while testing, chart this observation.
10. Wash hands and document the procedure.

CHARTING EXAMPLE

| 01/16/08 4:30 PM | Visual acuity OD 20/40–1 OS 20/20 with correction. Dr. Smart aware. |
| | ———————————— C. Mayers, CMA |

Procedure 6-9 Color Perception

Equipment
- Ishihara color plates

1. Put on gloves (to protect the plates) and get the Ishihara color plate book.
2. Seat the patient comfortably in a quiet, well-lighted room.
3. Instruct patients who wear glasses or contact lenses to keep them on.
4. Hold the first plate about 30 inches from the patient. Ask if he or she can see the number in the dots on the plate.
5. Record results by noting the number or figure the patient reports on each plate, using the plate number followed by the response.
6. If the patient cannot distinguish the pattern, record as the plate number followed by the letter X.
7. Record results for plates 1 to 10. Plate 11 requires the patient to trace the winding bluish-green line between the two X's. (Patients with a color deficit will not be able to trace the line.)
8. Store the book in a closed, protected area away from light.
9. Remove gloves and wash your hands.

Procedure 6-10 Eye Irrigation

Equipment
- Physician's order
- Patient record
- Small sterile basin if sterile solution is used
- Irrigating solution (water) and medication (if ordered)
- Protective barrier or towels
- Emesis basin
- Sterile bulb syringe
- Tissues

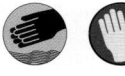

1. If medication is ordered, check the label three times and make sure it indicates ophthalmic use.

2. If both eyes are to be treated, use separate equipment (solution and bulb syringe) to avoid cross-contamination.
3. Position patient with the head tilted and affected eye lower, or lying with affected eye down; drape.
4. Place emesis basin against the upper cheek near the eye with towel underneath. With clean gauze, wipe eye from the inner canthus outward to remove debris from lashes.
5. Separate the lids with your thumb and forefinger.
6. Irrigate from inner to outer canthus, holding the syringe 1 inch above the eye. Use gentle pressure and do not touch the eye. The physician will order the time or amount of solution to be used.
7. Tissue off excess solution from the patient's face.
8. Dispose of or sanitize equipment.
9. Remove gloves and wash your hands.
10. Record the procedure.

Procedure 6-11 Ear Irrigation

Equipment
- Physician's order
- Patient's record
- Irrigating syringe or device
- Emesis or ear basin
- Waterproof barrier or towels
- Otoscope
- Irrigating solution (water)
- Bowl for solution
- Gauze

1. Position patient comfortably erect.
2. View affected ear with otoscope to locate the foreign matter or cerumen.

3. Straighten the ear canal (Fig. 6-2).
   • *Adults:* Pull pinna up and back.
   • *Children:* Pull pinna down and back.
4. Drape patient.
5. Tilt head toward the affected side.
6. Place basin under the affected ear.
7. Fill irrigating syringe or turn on irrigating device.
8. Gently position auricle as described.
9. Place tip of the syringe in the auditory meatus and direct solution flow gently up toward the roof of the canal.
10. Irrigate for the prescribed period or until the desired result (cerumen removal) is obtained.
11. If the patient complains of pain or discomfort, stop the irrigation and notify the physician.
12. Dry patient's external ear with gauze.
13. Have patient sit awhile with the affected ear down to drain solution.

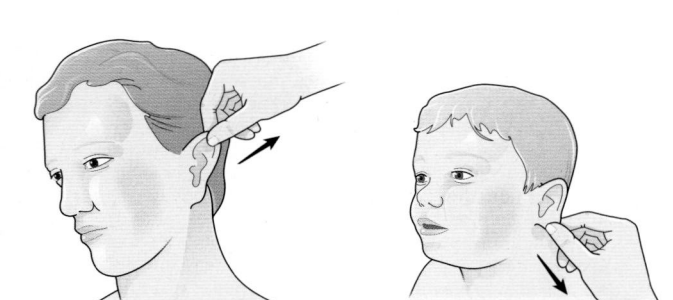

Figure 6-2. The shape of the ear canal changes with growth. To allow good inspection, position the ear as illustrated.

14. Inspect the ear with the otoscope to determine results.
15. Care for or dispose of equipment. Clean the work area.
16. Wash your hands.
17. Record the procedure.

03/17/08 **3:30 PM**	AD irrigated with 500 mL sterile water; return clear with 2 large pieces of yellow-brown cerumen noted.
	——————— S. Stark, CMA

WARNING ⚠

If the tympanic membrane appears perforated, do not irrigate without checking with the physician. Solution may be forced into the middle ear through the perforation.

Procedure 6-12 Audiometry Testing

Equipment
- Audiometer
- Otoscope

1. Using an otoscope or audioscope with a light source, visually inspect the ear canal and tympanic membrane.
2. If you see an obstruction (e.g., cerumen), notify the physician.

3. Choose the correct size tip for the end of the audiometer.
4. Attach a speculum to fit the patient's external auditory meatus, making sure the ear canal is occluded with the speculum in place.
5. With the speculum in the ear canal, retract the pinna (up and back for adults; down and back for children).
6. Turn the instrument on and select screening level. There is a pretest tone for practice if necessary.
7. Press the start button and observe the tone indicators and patient responses.
8. Screen the other ear.
9. If the patient fails to respond at any frequency, rescreening is required.
10. If the patient fails rescreening, notify the physician.
11. Record the results.

PULMONARY PROCEDURES

Procedure 6-13   Instruct a Patient on Using a Peak Flowmeter

Equipment
- Peak flowmeter
- Recording documentation form

1. Assemble the peak flowmeter, disposable mouthpiece, and patient documentation form.
2. Holding the peak flowmeter upright, explain how to read and reset the gauge after each reading.
3. Have patient put the peak flowmeter mouthpiece in the mouth, forming a tight seal with the lips.

4. Instruct patient to take a deep breath, then blow hard into the mouthpiece without blocking the back of the flowmeter.
5. Note the number on the flowmeter corresponding to the level at which the sliding gauge stopped after the patient blew into the mouthpiece. Reset the gauge to zero.
6. Instruct patient to perform this procedure three times consecutively, in the morning and at night, and to record the highest reading.
7. Explain how to clean the mouthpiece; instruct patient not to immerse flowmeter in water.
8. Document the procedure.

Procedure 6-14 Perform a Pulmonary Function Test

Equipment
- Physician's order
- Patient's medical record
- Spirometer and appropriate cables
- Calibration syringe and log book
- Disposable mouthpiece
- Printer
- Nose clip

1. Turn on the pulmonary function test machine.
2. If spirometer has not been calibrated per office policy, calibrate it using the calibration syringe following manufacturer's instructions. Record the calibration in the log book.
3. Attach the appropriate cable, tubing, and mouthpiece.
4. Using the machine keyboard, enter the patient's name or identification number, age, weight, height, sex, race, and smoking history.

5. Have patient remove any restrictive clothing (e.g., necktie).
6. Show patient how to apply the nose clip.
7. Have patient stand, breathe in deeply, and blow into the mouthpiece as hard as possible.
8. Coach patient as needed to obtain an adequate reading.
9. Continue the procedure until three adequate readings, or maneuvers, are performed. Print the results.
10. Care for equipment and dispose of mouthpiece in biohazard container.
11. Wash your hands.
12. Document the procedure. Place printed results in chart.

CHARTING EXAMPLE

06/12/08 **3:00 PM**	PFT performed for employment physical as ordered by Dr. John. ×3 maneuvers obtained without difficulty. Dr. John notified of results in chart.

——————————— P. Hill, CMA

WARNING❗

The patient may get dizzy or lightheaded during the procedure. Have chair available close by if the need arises.

TABLE **6-2**	Abnormal Breath Sounds
Breath Sound	Description
Bubbling	Gurgling sounds as air passes through moist secretions in airways.
Crackles (rales)	Crackling sound, usually inspiratory, as air passes through moist secretions in airways. Fine to medium crackles indicate secretions in small airways and alveoli. Medium to coarse crackles indicate secretions in larger airways.
Friction rub	Dry, rubbing, or grating sound.
Rhonchi	Low-pitched, continuous sound as air moves past thick mucus or narrowed air passages.
Stertor	Snoring sound on inspiration or expiration; indicates a partial airway obstruction.
Stridor	Shrill, harsh inspiratory sound; indicates laryngeal obstruction
Wheeze	High-pitched musical sound, either inspiratory or expiratory; indicates partial airway obstruction

CARDIAC PROCEDURES

Procedure 6-15 Perform a 12-Lead ECG

Equipment
- Physician's order
- Patient record
- ECG machine with cable and lead wires
- ECG paper
- Disposable electrodes that contain coupling gel
- Gown and drape
- Skin preparation materials, including razor and antiseptic wipes

1. Turn on the machine and enter patient's name and/or identification number, age, sex, height, weight, blood pressure, and medications.
2. Instruct patient to disrobe above the waist; provide gown for privacy. Female patients should remove nylons or tights.
3. Position patient supine; drape.
4. Prepare skin as needed. Wear gloves if shaving hair is necessary.
5. Apply electrodes snugly against the fleshy, muscular parts of the upper arms and lower legs according to the manufacturer's directions. Apply the chest electrodes, V_1–V_6 (Fig. 6-3).
6. Connect lead wires securely according to the color-coded notations on the connectors (RA, LA, RL, LL, V_1–V_6).
7. Determine the sensitivity, or gain, and paper speed settings on the ECG machine before running the test. Set sensitivity or gain on 1 and paper speed on 25 mm/second.
8. Depress the automatic button on the ECG machine to obtain the 12-lead tracing. The machine will automatically move from one lead to the next.

9. If the physician wants only a rhythm strip tracing, use the manual mode of operation and select the lead manually.
10. When tracing is complete and printed, check the ECG for artifacts and a standardization mark.
11. If tracing is adequate, turn off machine and remove and discard the electrodes.
12. Assist patient to sit and help with dressing if needed.
13. For a single-channel machine, roll the ECG strip to secure the roll. Do not fold the ECG tracing or apply clips.
14. Mount the ECG on 8×11 inch paper or a form before placing in chart.
15. Record the procedure.
16. Place ECG tracing and patient's chart on physician's desk, or give it directly to the physician, as instructed.

CHARTING EXAMPLE

06/12/08	Pre-employment 12-lead ECG obtained
9:45 AM	and placed in chart.

——————————— A. Perez, CMA

BOX 6-2 Abbreviations Used in Performing ECGs

RA	right arm
LA	left arm
LL	left leg
RL	right leg
V_1–V_6	chest leads
aVR	augmented voltage right arm
aVL	augmented voltage left arm
aVF	augmented voltage left foot or leg

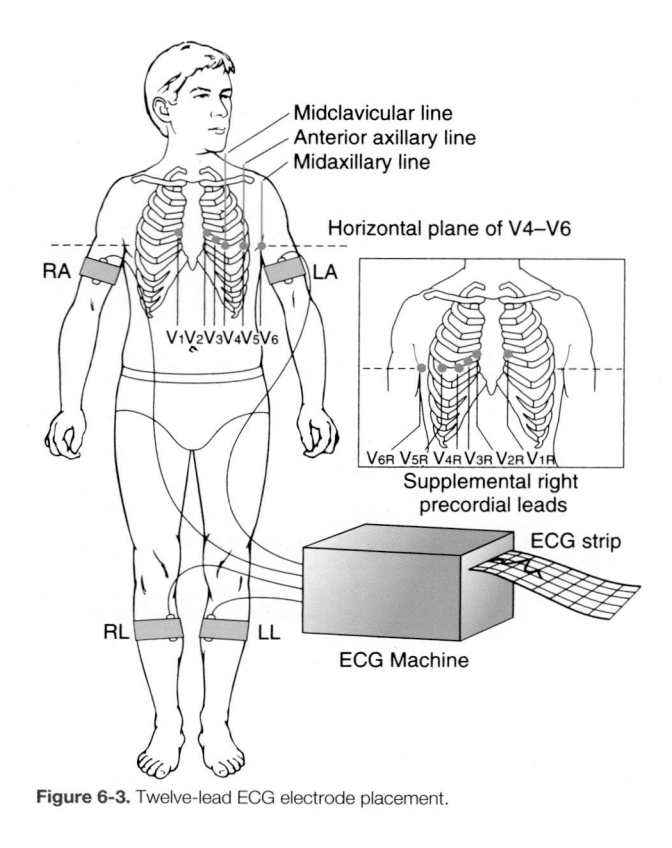

Figure 6-3. Twelve-lead ECG electrode placement.

BOX 6-3 Positioning of Unipolar Precordial (Chest) Leads

- $LV_1 = (RA + LA + LL)$ to V_1: Fourth intercostal space at right margin of sternum
- $LV_2 = (RA + LA + LL)$ to V_2: Fourth intercostal space at left margin of sternum
- $LV_3 = (RA + LA + LL)$ to V_3: Midway between V_2 and V_4
- $LV_4 = (RA + LA + LL)$ to V_4: Fifth intercostal space at junction of midclavicular line
- $LV_5 = (RA + LA + LL)$ to V_5: Horizontal level of V_4 at left anterior axillary line
- $V_6 = (RA + LA + LL)$ to V_6: Horizontal level of V_4 and V_5 at midaxillary line

Procedure 6-16 Apply a Holter Monitor

Equipment
- Physician's order
- Patient record
- Holter monitor with appropriate lead wires
- Fresh batteries
- Carrying case with strap
- Disposable electrodes with coupling gel
- Adhesive tape
- Gown and drape
- Skin preparation materials including a razor and antiseptic wipes
- Diary

Types of Artifacts

Artifact	Possible Cause	How to Prevent Problems
Wandering baseline	Electrodes too tight or too loose Electrolyte gel dried out Skin has oil, lotion, or excessive hair	Apply electrodes properly Apply new electrodes Prepare skin before applying electrodes
Muscle or somatic artifact	Patient cannot remain still because of tremors or fear	Reassure patient; explain procedure, stress the need to keep still, patients with disease may be unable to stay motionless
Alternating current	Improperly grounded ECG machine Electrical interference in room Dangling lead wires	Check cables to ensure properly grounded machine before beginning test Move patient or unplug appliances in immediate area Arrange wires along contours or patient's body.

WANDERING BASELINE

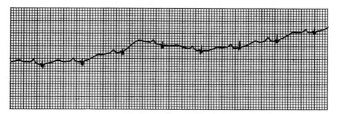

SOMATIC MUSCLE TREMOR

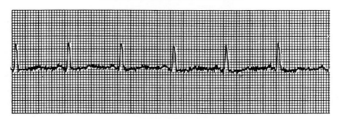

AC INTERFERENCE

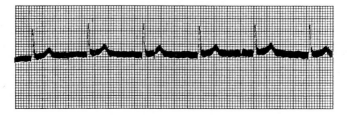

1. Remind patient to carry out all normal activities for the test duration.
2. Explain the incident diary's purpose; emphasize the need to carry it at all times.
3. Have patient disrobe from the waist up and put on gown; drape for privacy.
4. With the patient seated, prepare the skin for electrode attachment. Provide privacy. Shave the skin if necessary while wearing gloves and cleanse with antiseptic wipes.
5. Expose electrodes' adhesive backing and attach firmly following manufacturer's instructions. Apply electrodes at the specified sites (Fig. 6-4):
   (a) Right manubrium border
   (b) Left manubrium border
   (c) Right sternal border at the fifth rib
   (d) Fifth rib at the anterior axillary line
   (e) Right lower rib cage over the cartilage as a ground lead.

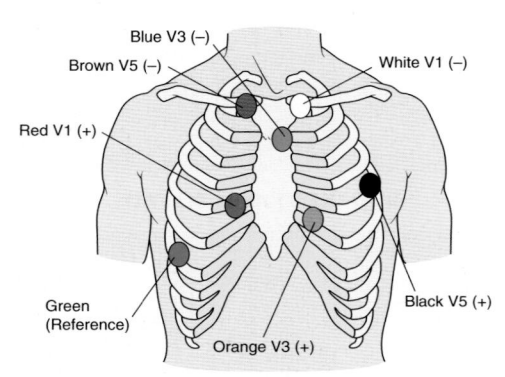

Figure 6-4. Sites for Holder electrodes.

6. Check that attachments are secure.
7. Position electrode connectors down toward the patient's feet. Attach the lead wires and secure with adhesive tape.
8. Connect the cable and run a baseline ECG by hooking the Holter to the ECG machine with the cable hookup.
9. Assist patient to dress carefully with the cable extending through the garment opening.
10. Plug the cable into recorder and mark diary. Give instructions for a return appointment to evaluate the recording and the diary.
11. Record the procedure.

PEDIATRIC PROCEDURES

Procedure 6-17 Infant Length and Weight

Equipment
- Examination table with clean paper
- Tape measure
- Infant scale
- Protective paper for the scale
- Growth chart

1. Ask parent to remove infant's clothing except for the diaper.
2. Place infant on examination table covered with clean paper. If using a measuring board, cover board with clean paper.
3. Fully extend infant's body. Hold the head in the midline and grasp the knees; press flat onto the table gently but firmly.

193

4. Mark the table paper with your pen at the top of the head and at the heel of the feet.
5. If you need assistance, ask the parent or a coworker to hold the child in position.
6. Measure between the marks; record the length on the growth chart and in the patient chart.
7. Carry the infant to the scale (or have the parent do so).
8. Place protective paper on the scale and balance the scale.
9. Remove the diaper, then place the infant on the scale. Keep one of your hands over or near the infant at all times.
10. Quickly move the counterweights to balance the apparatus.
11. Pick up the infant and have the parent replace diaper.
12. Record the weight on the growth chart and in the patient chart.

Procedure 6-18 Infant Head and Chest Circumference

Equipment
• Paper or cloth measuring tape
• Growth chart

1. Place infant supine on examination table or ask parent to hold child.
2. Measure around the head above the eyebrow and posteriorly at the largest part of the occiput. For an accurate reading, measure the largest circumference.
3. Record head circumference on the growth chart and in the patient chart.
4. With clothing removed from the chest, measure around the infant's chest at the nipple line. Keep measuring tape at the same level anterior and posterior.
5. Record chest circumference on the growth chart and in the patient chart.

Procedure 6-19 Apply a Pediatric Urine Collection Device

Equipment
- Personal antiseptic wipes
- Pediatric urine collection bag
- Completed laboratory request slip
- Biohazard transport container

1. Place child supine. Ask parent to help as needed.
2. Put on gloves.
3. Clean the genitalia:
   (a) *Girls:* Cleanse front to back with separate wipes for each downward stroke on the outer labia. Use last clean wipe between the inner labia.
   (b) *Boys:* Retract foreskin if child is uncircumcised. Cleanse the meatus in an ever-widening circle. Discard wipe and repeat the procedure. Return foreskin to its proper position.
4. Holding collection device, remove upper portion of the paper backing and press it around the mons pubis. Remove the second section and press it against perineum.
5. Loosely attach diaper.
6. Give child fluids unless contraindicated and check diaper frequently.
7. When child has voided, remove the device, clean residual adhesive from skin, and put on clean diaper.
8. Prepare specimen for transport to laboratory or process it appropriately.
9. Remove gloves and wash your hands.
10. Record the procedure.

TABLE **6-3** Normal Pulse Rates for Children	
Age	Rate/Minute
Newborn	100–180
3 mo–2 yr	80–150
2–10 yr	65–130
10 yr and older	60–100

TABLE **6-4** Normal Respiratory Rates for Children	
Age	Rate/Minute
Newborn	30–35
1–2 yr	25–30
4–6 yr	23–25
8 yr and older	16–20

TABLE **6-5**	Normal Blood Pressure for Children		
Age	Systolic	Diastolic
Newborn	<90	<70
1–5 yr	<110	<70
10 yr and older	<120	<84

In millimeters of mecury.

OTHER SPECIALTY PROCEDURES

Procedure 6-20 Apply a Tubular Gauze Bandage

Equipment
- Tubular gauze
- Applicator
- Tape
- Scissors

1. Choose the appropriate size tubular gauze applicator and gauze width according to the size of the area to be covered. (Check manufacturer's supply charts.)
2. Cut adhesive tape in lengths to secure the gauze ends.
3. Place gauze bandage on the applicator as follows:
   (a) Place applicator upright (open end up) on a flat surface.

(b) Pull a sufficient length of gauze from the stock box; do not cut it yet.

(c) Open the end of the length of gauze and slide it over the upper end of the applicator. Estimate and push the amount of gauze that will be needed for this procedure onto the applicator.

(d) Cut gauze when the required amount is transferred to the applicator.

4. Place applicator over the distal end of the affected part and apply the gauze by pulling it over the applicator onto the skin. Hold it in place as you move to step 5.

5. Slide applicator up to the proximal end of the affected part. Hold the gauze at the proximal end of the affected part and pull applicator and gauze toward the distal end.

6. Continue holding gauze in place at the proximal end. Pull applicator 1 to 2 inches past the end of the affected part.

7. Turn applicator one full turn to anchor the bandage.

8. Move applicator toward the proximal part as before.

9. Move applicator forward about 1 inch beyond the original starting point. Anchor the bandage again.

10. Repeat procedure until desired coverage is obtained. The final layer should end at the proximal part of the affected area. Cut any extra gauze from the applicator. Remove the applicator.

11. Secure the bandage with adhesive tape, or cut gauze into two tails and tie them around the closest proximal joint.

12. Care for or dispose of equipment. Clean the work area.

13. Wash your hands and record the procedure.

Procedure 6-21 Assist with Colon Procedures

Equipment
- Appropriate instrument (flexible or rigid sigmoidoscope, anoscope, or proctoscope)
- Water-soluble lubricant
- Gown and drape
- Cotton swabs

- Suction (if not part of the scope)
- Biopsy forceps
- Specimen container with preservative
- Completed laboratory requisition form
- Personal wipes or tissues
- Equipment for assessing vital signs

1. Write patient's name on specimen container label and complete laboratory requisition.
2. Ensure equipment is in working order. Check light source on flexible sigmoidoscope.
3. Inform patient that a sensation of pressure or need to defecate may be felt during the procedure and that the pressure is from the instrument and will ease. The patient may also feel gas pressure when air is insufflated during sigmoidoscopy. *Note:* The patient may have been ordered to take a mild sedative before the procedure.
4. Instruct patient to empty the bladder.
5. Assess vital signs; record.
6. Have patient disrobe from the waist down and put on a gown; drape.
7. Assist patient onto the examination table. If the instrument is an anoscope or a fiberoptic device, Sims' position or a side-lying position is most comfortable. If a rigid instrument is used, the patient will assume a knee-chest position or be placed on a proctology table that supports the patient in a knee-chest position. *Note:* Do not ask the patient to assume the knee-chest position until the physician is ready to begin. The position is difficult to maintain. Drape the patient.
8. Assist physician as needed with lubricant, instruments, power, swabs, suction, and specimen containers.

9. During the procedure, monitor the patient's response and offer reassurance. Instruct the patient to breathe slowly through pursed lips to aid in relaxation if necessary.
10. When the physician is finished, assist the patient into a comfortable position and allow a rest period. Offer personal cleaning wipes or tissues. Take the vital signs before allowing the patient to stand and assist the patient from the table and with dressing as needed. Give the patient any instructions regarding care after the procedure and follow-up as ordered by the physician.
11. Clean the room and route the specimen to the laboratory with the requisition. Disinfect or dispose of the supplies.
12. Wash your hands and record the procedure.

WARNING ⚠

Colon examination procedures may cause cardiac arrhythmias and a change in blood pressure. Carefully monitor patient response during the procedure. Alert the physician if the patient seems distressed.

Procedure 6-22 Male Urinary Catheterization

Equipment
- Sterile straight catheterization tray with 14 or 16 French catheter
- Sterile gloves
- Antiseptic solution
- Sterile specimen cup with lid
- Lubricant
- Sterile drape
- Patient gown and drape for privacy
- Examination light

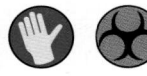

1. Have patient disrobe from waist down; provide gown and drape.
2. Place patient supine.
3. Open tray and place it to the patient's side on the examination table or on top of the patient's thighs.
4. Put on sterile gloves.
5. Place sterile drape under the glans penis.
6. Open antiseptic swabs and place them upright inside the catheter tray.
7. Open lubricant and squeeze a generous amount onto the tip of the catheter as it lies in the bottom of the catheter tray.
8. Place sterile urine specimen cup and lid to the side of the tray.
9. With nondominant hand, pick up the penis, exposing the urinary meatus. This hand is now contaminated and must not be moved out of position until the catheter is inserted into the urinary bladder.
10. Cleanse the urinary meatus using the antiseptic swabs by wiping from top to bottom on each side and down the middle of the exposed urinary meatus. Use a separate swab for each side and the middle (Fig. 6-5).
11. With sterile dominant hand, insert lubricated catheter tip into the urinary meatus approximately 4 to 6 inches. Leave the other end of the catheter in the tray, which will collect the urine.
12. When urine begins to flow, hold the catheter in position with nondominant hand. Use dominant hand to direct urine flow into the specimen cup, if needed.
13. When urine flow has slowed or stopped *or* 1000 mL has been obtained, carefully pull catheter straight out.
14. Wipe the glans penis with drape.
15. Dispose of urine, catheter, tray, and supplies in biohazard container.
16. If a urine specimen was obtained, label the container and complete the laboratory requisition. Process the specimen appropriately.
17. Remove gloves and wash your hands.

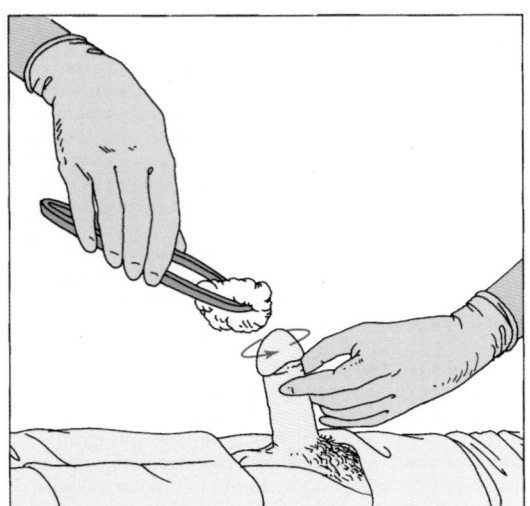

Figure 6-5. Expose the urinary meatus and cleanse from top to bottom.

18. Instruct the patient to dress and give any follow-up information.
19. Document the procedure.

Procedure 6-23 Female Urinary Catheterization

Equipment
- Sterile straight catheterization tray with 14 or 16 French catheter
- Sterile gloves
- Antiseptic solution

- Sterile specimen cup with lid
- Lubricant, sterile drape
- Examination light
- Patient gown and drape for privacy

1. Have patient disrobe from waist down; provide gown and drape.
2. Place patient in dorsal recumbent or lithotomy position.
3. Open tray and place it between the patient's legs.
4. Shine examination light on the perineum.
5. Put on sterile gloves.
6. Place sterile drape under the buttocks.
7. Open antiseptic swabs and place them upright inside the catheter tray.
8. Open lubricant and squeeze a generous amount onto the tip of the catheter as it lies in the catheter tray.
9. Place sterile urine specimen cup and lid to the side of the tray.
10. With nondominant hand, spread the labia to expose the urinary meatus. This hand is now contaminated and must not be moved out of position until the catheter is in the bladder.
11. Cleanse the urinary meatus using the antiseptic swabs by wiping from top to bottom on each side and down the middle of the exposed urinary meatus. Use a separate swab for each side and the middle (Fig. 6-6).
12. With sterile dominant hand, insert lubricated catheter tip into the urinary meatus approximately 3 inches. Leave the other end of the catheter in the tray, which will collect the urine.

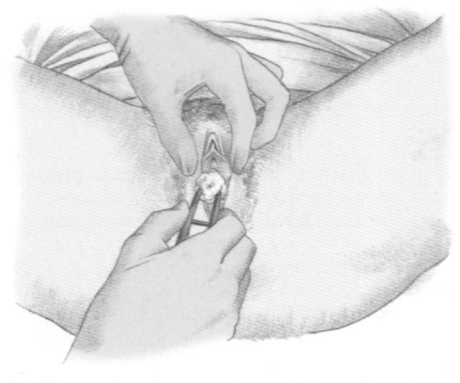

Figure 6-6. Expose the urinary meatus and cleanse from top to bottom.

13. When urine begins to flow, hold the catheter in position with nondominant hand. Use dominant hand to direct urine flow into specimen cup if needed.
14. When urine flow has slowed or stopped *or* 1000 mL has been obtained, carefully pull catheter straight out.
15. Wipe the perineum with drape.
16. Dispose of urine, catheter, tray, and supplies in biohazard container.
17. If a urine specimen was obtained, label the container and complete the laboratory requisition. Process the specimen appropriately.
18. Remove gloves and wash your hands.
19. Instruct the patient to dress and give any follow-up information.
20. Document the procedure.

02/14/08	Catheterization with a 14-fr straight cath,
9:15 AM	300 mL dark amber urine obtained,
	specimen to Acme lab for C&S.
	——————————— S. Strobb, CMA

Procedure 6-24   Assist with the Pelvic Examination and Pap Smear

Equipment
- Gown and drape
- Vaginal speculum
- Cotton-tipped applicators
- Water-soluble lubricant
- Examination light
- Tissues
- Pap smear materials
- Cervical spatula and/or brush, glass slides and fixative solution *or* container with liquid medium to preserve the cells
- Laboratory request form
- Identification labels
- Other materials that may be required by laboratory

1. Label slides with specimen date and type. For liquid medium, label outside of the container.
2. Ask the patient to empty her bladder and if necessary collect a urine specimen.

205

3. Provide a gown and drape and ask patient to disrobe from the waist down.
4. Position in dorsal lithotomy position with patient's buttocks at the bottom edge of the table.
5. Adjust drape to cover abdomen and knees, exposing the genitalia.
6. Adjust the light over genitalia for maximum visibility.
7. Assist physician as needed by handing instruments and supplies.
8. Put on gloves and hold microscope slides or container of liquid medium while physician obtains the specimen.
9. For glass slides, spray or cover with fixative solution.
10. When physician removes vaginal speculum, receive it in basin or other container.
11. Apply lubricant across physician's two gloved fingers.
12. Encourage patient to relax during bimanual examination as needed.
13. When examination is finished, help patient slide up to the top of the examination table and remove feet from stirrups.
14. Offer tissues to remove excess lubricant.
15. Help patient sit if necessary; watch for signs of vertigo.
16. Provide privacy as patient dresses.
17. Reinforce physician instructions regarding follow-up appointments.
18. Advise the patient on obtaining laboratory findings from the Pap smear.
19. Care for or dispose of equipment. Clean the examination room.
20. Wash your hands.
21. Document your responsibilities during the procedure.

TABLE 6-6	Classifications of Papanicolaou Tests
Class	Characteristics
I	Normal test, no atypical cells
II	Atypical cells but no evidence of malignancy
III	Atypical cells possible but not conclusive for malignancy
IV	Cells strongly suggest malignancy
V	Strong evidence of malignancy

Emergency Procedures

7

BOX 7-1 Signs and Symptoms of Shock

- Low blood pressure
- Restlessness or signs of fear
- Thirst
- Nausea
- Cool, clammy skin
- Pale skin with cyanosis (bluish color) at the lips and earlobes
- Rapid and weak pulse

Procedure 7-1 Administer Oxygen

Equipment
- Oxygen tank with regulator
- Oxygen delivery system (nasal cannula, mask)

1. Check physician's order for oxygen amount and delivery method.
2. Connect distal end of tubing on cannula or mask to adapter on oxygen tank regulator.

3. Place nasal cannula into the nares, or secure mask over the nose and mouth.
4. Turn regulator dial to the ordered number of liters per minute.
5. Record the procedure.

CHARTING EXAMPLE

12/23/08 **2:15 PM**	Oxygen applied per nasal cannula at 4L/min as ordered.
	———————————— J. Leigh, CMA

Procedure 7-2 Perform CPR (Adult)

Equipment
- Mouth-to-mouth barrier device
- Gloves

1. Determine unresponsiveness. Shake patient and shout "Are you okay?"
2. If patient is unresponsive, assess airway patency and respirations using the head-tilt, chin-lift maneuver with patient supine (Fig. 7-1).
3. Instruct coworker to get the physician and emergency medical cart.
4. Put on gloves.
5. Open the airway and assess for breathing.
6. If breathing is adequate, place patient in recovery position (side-lying) until the patient regains consciousness or the physician instructs you to call EMS.

209

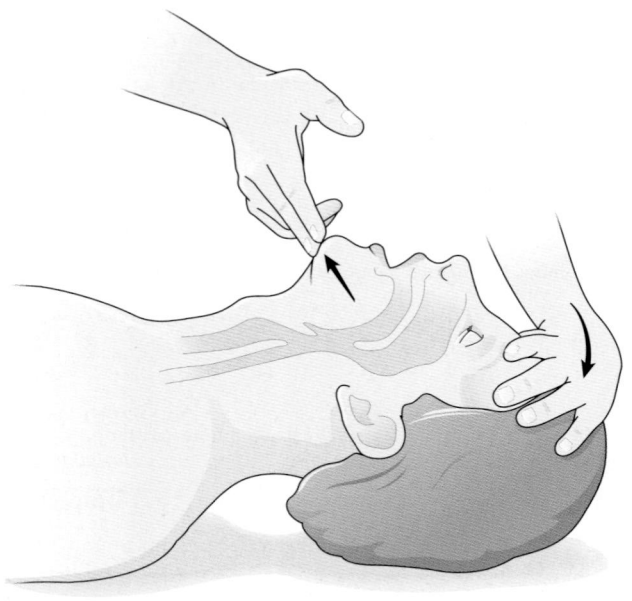

Figure 7-1. The head-tilt, chin-lift technique for opening the airway. The head is tilted backward with one hand *(down arrow)* while the fingers of the other hand lift the chin forward *(up arrow)*.

7. If breathing is not adequate, begin rescue breathing.
8. After giving two breaths, check carotid pulse.
9. If pulse is present but breathing is inadequate, continue rescue breathing.
10. If adequate breathing resumes, place patient in recovery position.
11. If no pulse is present, follow protocol for chest compressions according to the standards of the training provided by the American Heart Association, the American Red Cross, or the National Safety Council.

12. Check carotid pulse after 1 minute of chest compressions.
13. If no pulse is present, continue chest compressions and rescue breathing. If pulse returns but respirations do not, continue rescue breathing.
14. Continue CPR until relieved by another health care provider or EMS arrives.

Procedure 7-3 Use an Automatic External Defibrillator (AED) (Adult)

Equipment
- Automatic external defibrillator
- Chest pads with connection cables appropriate for the AED machine
- Scissors
- Dry gauze pads
- Gloves

1. Determine unresponsiveness. Shake the patient and shout "Are you okay?"
2. If patient is unresponsive, assess airway patency and respirations, giving two rescue breaths and checking for the presence of a carotid pulse (see Procedure 7-2).
3. Instruct coworker to notify the physician and obtain the emergency cart and AED.
4. Begin CPR if there is no pulse or adequate respirations.
5. Continue CPR while a second rescuer removes the patient's shirt and prepares the chest for the AED electrodes. This second rescuer will operate the AED.
6. Place AED pads on the upper and lower right chest.
7. Connect the wire from the electrodes to the AED unit and turn it on.
8. Follow directions given by the AED. Do not touch the patient.
   (a) If electrical shock is not indicated, the AED will say this and instruct you to resume CPR.

211

(b) If electrical shock is indicated, the second rescuer delivers it.

9. Continue following directions given by the AED, which will include either re-shocking the patient or resuming CPR. Always assess respirations and carotid pulse before resuming CPR.

10. Continue this pattern until EMS arrives and takes over the emergency procedure.

Procedure 7-4   Manage a Foreign Body Airway Obstruction (Adult)

Equipment
- Mouth-to-mouth barrier device
- Gloves

1. *If the patient is conscious:* Ask "Are you choking?"
   If patient can speak or cough, observe the patient for increased distress and assist as needed. Do not perform abdominal thrusts.

2. *If the patient cannot speak or cough and displays the universal distress sign:* Perform abdominal thrusts and have a coworker notify the physician:
   (a) Stand behind the patient and wrap your arms around the waist.
   (b) Make a fist with your nondominant hand, thumb side against the patient's abdomen.
   (c) Grasp your fist with your dominant hand and give quick upward thrusts.
   (d) Relax your arms between each thrust and make each thrust forceful enough to dislodge the obstruction in the airway.

    (e) Repeat thrusts until the object is expelled and the patient can breathe or the patient becomes unconscious.
3. *If the patient is unconscious or becomes unconscious:* Apply gloves and perform a tongue-jaw lift followed by a finger sweep to try to remove the object.
4. Open the airway and try to give the patient two rescue breaths (see Procedure 7-2).
5. If rescue breaths are obstructed, begin abdominal thrusts:
    (a) Straddle the patient's hips.
    (b) Place the palm of one hand between the patient's navel and the xiphoid process.
    (c) Lace your fingers with the other hand against the back of the properly positioned hand.
6. Give five abdominal thrusts then repeat the tongue-jaw lift and finger sweep maneuver.
7. Attempt to give rescue breaths.
    (a) If rescue breaths adequately ventilate the patient, continue until the patient resumes breathing *or* EMS arrives.
    (b) While performing rescue breathing, periodically check for a carotid pulse; be prepared to start CPR.
8. If no object is removed or the lungs cannot be inflated, continue the cycle of abdominal thrusts, tongue-jaw lift, finger sweep, and rescue breaths until EMS arrives.

WARNING❗

- Give obese or pregnant patients chest thrusts rather than abdominal thrusts.
- Consider children over 8 years to be adults for the purpose of foreign body airway obstruction.

Procedure 7-5 Control Bleeding

Equipment
- Gloves
- Sterile gauze pads

1. Determine what caused the bleeding, if possible.
2. Take the patient to examination room and have someone notify the physician.
3. Apply gloves and open 2 to 3 packages of sterile 4 × 4 gauze pads.
4. Have the patient lie down on the exam table.
5. Apply direct pressure to the wound with gauze pads until bleeding stops. Hold pressure for at least 20 minutes.
6. If bleeding continues or seeps through the gauze, apply additional gauze while continuing direct pressure.
7. If directed by physician, apply direct pressure to the artery delivering blood to the area while continuing direct pressure to the wound.
8. When the bleeding is controlled, assist the physician with a minor office surgical procedure to close the wound *or* notify EMS for transport to the hospital.
9. Monitor for signs of shock.

WARNING

Do not remove saturated pressure dressings. Doing so disrupts the clotting process and renews bleeding. Reinforce dressings without disturbing the site.

Procedure 7-6   Manage a Patient with a Diabetic Emergency

Equipment
- Blood glucose monitor and strips
- Fruit juice or oral glucose tablets
- Glucometer, strips, lancet, gauze pads, and alcohol swabs

1. Escort patient into the examination room.
2. Determine if the patient is a known diabetic.
3. Determine if the patient has eaten or taken any medication.
4. Notify the physician.
5. Perform a capillary stick for a blood glucose test.
6. Give test results to the physician and treat the patient as ordered.
   (a) *Hyperglycemia:* Administer insulin subcutaneously.
   (b) *Hypoglycemia:* Administer a quick-acting sugar, such as an oral glucose tablet or fruit juice.
7. Notify EMS as instructed by the physician if the symptoms do not improve or worsen.
8. Document any observations and treatments given.

BOX 7-2 **Signs and Symptoms of Hyperglycemia and Hypoglycemia**

Hyperglycemia
* Flushed, dry skin
* A sweet, fruity smell on the breath
* Thirst
* Deep respirations
* Rapid, weak pulse
* Abdominal pain

Hypoglycemia
* Pale, moist skin
* Shallow, fast respirations
* Rapid, bounding pulse
* Weakness
* Shakiness

BOX 7-3 **Emergency Care for Fractures**

- Assume that an injured limb is fractured until proven otherwise.
- Assess the patient; record pulse, temperature, and sensation beyond the injury.
- Splint injured limb without altering the position.
- Handle the site as little as possible to avoid further injury.
- Splint the joints above and below the injury to immobilize the area.
- Transport to the nearest emergency room or x-ray facility according to the physician orders.
- Document the injury and treatment given in the medical record

BOX 7-4 **Emergency Care for Burns**

- Assess the situation for danger to you, then remove burn source.
- Assess the patient for response, airway, and pulse.
- Wrap the patient in a clean, dry sheet if burn is extensive. Cover small areas with nonadherent gauze.
- Administer oxygen.
- Keep the patient warm and transport as quickly as possible according to physician instructions.
- Document the injury and treatment given in the medical record

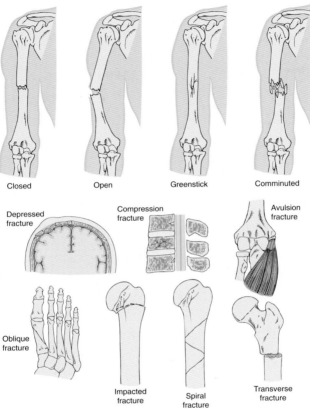

Figure 7-2. Types of fractures.

Closed

Open

Greenstick

Comminuted

Depressed fracture

Compression fracture

Avulsion fracture

Oblique fracture

Impacted fracture

Spiral fracture

Transverse fracture

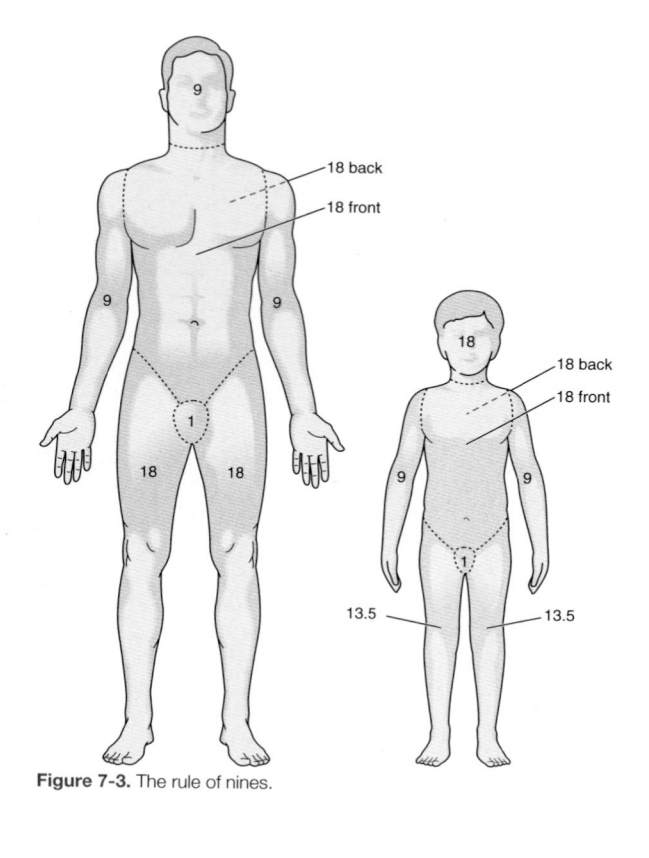

Figure 7-3. The rule of nines.

Procedure 7-7 Caring for a Patient During a Seizure

1. Help the patient to the floor.
2. Protect the head and limbs.
3. Provide privacy.
4. Alert the physician.
5. When seizure is over, place patient in side-lying position.

WARNING❗
Do not put anything in the patient's mouth.

Tools

8

HIPAA

The Health Insurance Portability and Accountability Act of 1996 is a federal law that requires all health care settings to ensure privacy and security of patient information.

HIPAA and Patients' Rights

Through HIPPA, the federal government recognizes that it is ethical to give patients certain rights. HIPAA protects the rights of patients by allowing them to:

- Ask to see and get a copy of their health records.
- Have corrections added to their health information.
- Receive a notice that tells how their health information may be used and shared.
- Decide if they want to give permission before their health information can be used or shared for certain purposes, such as for marketing.
- Get a report on when and why their health information was shared for certain purposes.
- If patients believe their rights have been denied or their health information is not being protected, they can file a complaint with the provider or health insurer.
- File a complaint with the U.S. government.

Patients can learn about their rights, including how to file a complaint, from the website at www.hhs.gov/ocr/hipaa/ or by calling 1-866-627-7748.

A Proper Authorization for Release of Information

I,_____, give my permission for _____ to release information generated in my medical record between the dates of _____ and _____ to _____.

Signature_____ Date_____
Witness_____ Date_____

Or

I,_____, give my permission for _____ to release information in my medical record regarding the care and treatment of _____ to _____.

Signature_____ Date_____
Witness_____ Date_____

Internet Resources for HIPAA Information

U.S. Department of Health and Human Services, CMS, HIPAA—General Information: http://www.cms.hhs.gov/HIPAAGenInfo/

U.S. Department of Health and Human Services, Office for Civil Rights, HIPAA—for HIPAA Privacy What's New items: http://www.hhs.gov/ocr/whatsnew.html

U.S. Department of Health and Human Services, Office of the Assistant Secretary for Planning and Evaluation—HIPAA administrative simplification requirements: http://aspe.os.dhhs.gov/admnsimp/

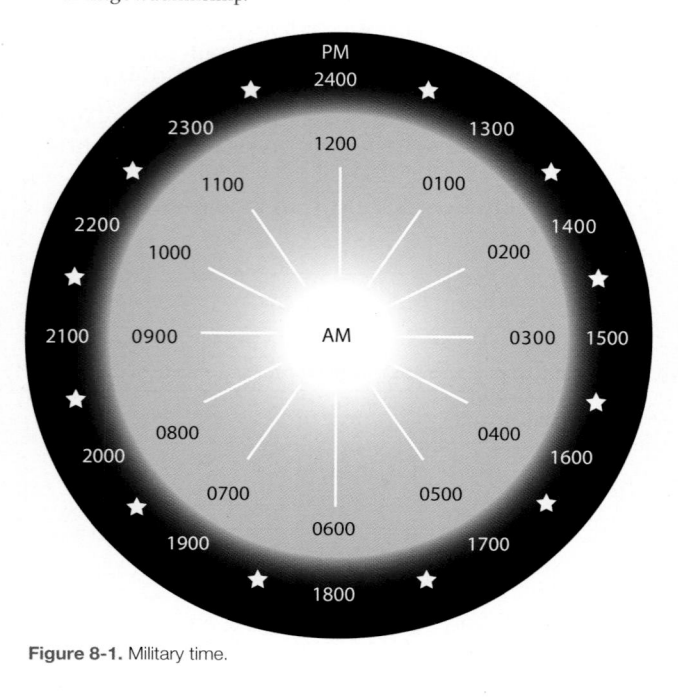

Figure 8-1. Military time.

TABLE 8-1	Disinfection Methods, Uses, and Precautions
Method	Uses and Precautions
Alcohol (70% isopropyl)	Used for noncritical items (countertops, glass thermometers, stethoscopes) Flammable; damages some rubber, plastic, and lenses
Chlorine (sodium hypochlorite or bleach)	Dilute 1:10 (1 part bleach to 10 parts water) Used for a broad spectrum of microbes Inexpensive and fast acting Corrosive, inactivated by organic matter, relatively unstable
Formaldehyde	Disinfectant and sterilant Regulated by OSHA Warnings must be marked on all containers and storage areas
Glutaraldehyde	Alkaline or acid Effective against bacteria, viruses, fungi, and some spores OSHA regulated; requires adequate ventilation, covered pans, gloves, masks Must display biohazard or chemical label

TABLE 8-1	Disinfection Methods, Uses, and Precautions (Continued)

Method	Uses and Precautions
Hydrogen peroxide	Stable and effective when used on inanimate objects Attacks membrane lipids, DNA, and other essential cell components Can damage plastic, rubber, and some metals
Iodine or iodophors	Bacteriostatic agent Not to be used on instruments May cause staining
Phenols (tuberculocidal)	Used for environmental items and equipment Requires gloves and eye protection Can cause skin irritation and burns

DNA, deoxyribonucleic acid; OSHA, Occupational Safety and Health Administration.

BOX 8-1 Abbreviations Commonly Used in Documentation

Abbreviations and symbols that appear in red font are considered "Dangerous Abbreviations" and should not be used.

Abbreviation or Symbol	Meaning
ā	before
A	anterior; assessment
A&P	auscultation and percussion
A&W	alive and well
AB	abortion
ABG	arterial blood gas
a.c.	before meals
ACE	angiotensin-converting enzyme
ACS	acute coronary syndrome
ACTH	adrenocorticotropic hormone
AD	right ear
ad lib.	as desired
ADH	antidiuretic hormone
ADHD	attention-deficit/hyperactivity disorder
AIDS	acquired immunodeficiency syndrome
AKA	above-knee amputation
alb	albumin
ALS	amyotrophic lateral sclerosis
ALT	alanine aminotransferase (enzyme)
a.m.	morning
amt	amount
ANS	autonomic nervous system
AP	anterior-posterior
APKD	adult polycystic kidney disease
Aq	water
AS	left ear
ASD	atrial septal defect
AST	aspartate aminotransferase (enzyme)

225

BOX 8-1 Abbreviations Commonly Used in Documentation (*Cont.*)

Abbreviation or Symbol	Meaning
AU	both ears
AV	atrioventricular
Ⓑ	bilateral
BAEP	brainstem auditory evoked potential
BAER	brainstem auditory evoked response
BCC	basal cell carcinoma
BD	bipolar disorder
b.i.d.	twice a day
BKA	below-knee amputation
BM	bowel movement
BMP	basic metabolic panel
BP	blood pressure
BPH	benign prostatic hypertrophy; benign prostatic hyperplasia
BRP	bathroom privileges
BS	blood sugar
BUN	blood urea nitrogen
Bx	biopsy
c̄	with
C	Celsius; centigrade
C&S	culture and sensitivity
CABG	coronary artery bypass graft
CAD	coronary artery disease
Cap	capsule
CAT	computed axial tomography
CBC	complete blood count
cc	cubic centimeter
CC	chief complaint
CCU	coronary (cardiac) care unit
CF	cystic fibrosis
CHF	congestive heart failure

BOX 8-1 Abbreviations Commonly Used in Documentation (*Cont.*)

Abbreviation or Symbol	Meaning
CIN	cervical intraepithelial neoplasia
CIS	carcinoma in situ
cm	centimeter
CMP	comprehensive metabolic panel
CNS	central nervous system
c/o	complains of
CO	cardiac output
CO_2	carbon dioxide
COPD	chronic obstructive pulmonary disease
CP	cerebral palsy; chest pain
CPAP	continuous positive airway pressure
CPD	cephalopelvic disproportion
CPR	cardiopulmonary resuscitation
CSF	cerebrospinal fluid
CSII	continuous subcutaneous insulin infusion
CT	computed tomography
CTA	computed tomographic angiography
cu mm or mm^3	cubic millimeter
CVA	cerebrovascular accident
CVS	chorionic villus sampling
CXR	chest x-ray
d	day
D&C	dilation and curettage
D&E	dilation and evacuation
DC	discharge; discontinue; doctor of chiropractic
DDS	doctor of dental surgery
DJD	degenerative joint disease
DKA	diabetic ketoacidosis
DO	doctor of osteopathy

BOX 8-1 Abbreviations Commonly Used in Documentation (*Cont.*)

Abbreviation or Symbol	Meaning
DPM	doctor of podiatric medicine
dr	dram
DRE	digital rectal exam
DTR	deep tendon reflex
DVT	deep vein thrombosis
Dx	diagnosis
ECG	electrocardiogram
echo	echocardiogram
ECT	electroconvulsive therapy
ECU	emergency care unit
ED	erectile dysfunction
EDC	estimated date of confinement
EDD	estimated date of delivery
EEG	electroencephalogram
EGD	esophagogastroduodenoscopy
EKG	electrocardiogram
EMG	electromyogram
ENT	ear, nose, and throat
EPS	electrophysiologic study
ER	emergency room
ERCP	endoscopic retrograde cholangiopancreatography
ESR	erythrocyte sedimentation rate
ESWL	extracorporeal shock wave lithotripsy
ETOH	ethyl alcohol
EUS	endoscopic ultrasonography
F	Fahrenheit
FBS	fasting blood sugar
Fe	iron
FH	family history
fl oz	fluid ounce

BOX 8-1   **Abbreviations Commonly Used in Documentation (*Cont.*)**

Abbreviation or Symbol	Meaning
FS	frozen section
FSH	follicle-stimulating hormone
Fx	fracture
g	gram
GAD	generalized anxiety disorder
GERD	gastroesophageal reflux disease
GH	growth hormone
GI	gastrointestinal
gm	gram
gr	grain
gt	drop
gtt	drops
GTT	glucose tolerance test
GYN	gynecology
h	hour
H&H	hemoglobin and hematocrit
H&P	history and physical
HAV	hepatitis A virus
HBV	hepatitis B virus
HCT or Hct	hematocrit
HCV	hepatitis C virus
HD	Huntington disease
HEENT	head, eyes, ears, nose, and throat
HGB or Hgb	hemoglobin
HIV	human immunodeficiency virus
hpf	high-power field
HPI	history of present illness
HPV	human papillomavirus
HRT	hormone replacement therapy
h.s.	hour of sleep
HSV-1	herpes simplex virus type 1

| BOX 8-1 | Abbreviations Commonly Used in Documentation (*Cont.*) |

Abbreviation or Symbol	Meaning
HSV-2	herpes simplex virus type 2
Ht	height
HTN	hypertension
Hx	history
I&D	incision and drainage
ICD	implantable cardioverter defibrillator
ICU	intensive care unit
ID	intradermal
IM	intramuscular
IMP	impression
IOL	intraocular lens
IP	inpatient
IUD	intrauterine device
IV	intravenous
IVP	intravenous pyelogram
IVU	intravenous urogram
JCAHO	Joint Commission on Accreditation of Healthcare Organizations
kg	kilogram
KUB	kidneys, ureters, bladder
L	liter
Ⓛ	left
L&W	living and well
LASIK	laser-assisted in situ keratomileusis
lb	pound
LEEP	loop electrosurgical excision procedure
LH	luteinizing hormone
LLETZ	large-loop excision of transformation zone
LLQ	left lower quadrant
LP	lumbar puncture

BOX 8-1 Abbreviations Commonly Used in Documentation (*Cont.*)

Abbreviation or Symbol	Meaning
lpf	low-power field
LTB	laryngotracheobronchitis
LUQ	left upper quadrant
m	meter
ⓜ	murmur
MCH	mean corpuscular (cell) hemoglobin
MCHC	mean corpuscular (cell) hemoglobin concentration
MCV	mean corpuscular (cell) volume
MRSA	methicillin resistant Staphylococcus aureus
MD	medical doctor; muscular dystrophy
mg	milligram
MI	myocardial infarction
ml or mL	milliliter
mm	millimeter
mm^3 or cu mm	cubic millimeter
MPI	myocardial perfusion image
MRA	magnetic resonance angiography
MRI	magnetic resonance imaging
MS	multiple sclerosis; musculoskeletal
MSH	melanocyte-stimulating hormone
MUGA	multiple-gated acquisition (scan)
MVP	mitral valve prolapse
NAD	no acute distress
NCV	nerve conduction velocity
NG	nasogastric
NK	natural killer (cell)
NKA	no known allergy
NKDA	no known drug allergy
noc.	night
NPO	nothing by mouth
NSAID	nonsteroidal antiinflammatory drug

BOX 8-1 Abbreviations Commonly Used in Documentation (*Cont.*)

Abbreviation or Symbol	Meaning
NSR	normal sinus rhythm
O	objective
O_2	oxygen
OA	osteoarthritis
OB	obstetrics
OCD	obsessive-compulsive disorder
OCP	oral contraceptive pill
OD	right eye; doctor of optometry
OH	occupational history
OP	outpatient
OR	operating room
ORIF	open reduction, internal fixation
OS	left eye
OU	both eyes
oz	ounce
p̄	after
P	plan; posterior; pulse
PA	posterior-anterior
PACU	postanesthetic care unit
$PaCO_2$	partial pressure of carbon dioxide
PaO_2	partial pressure of oxygen
Pap	Papanicolaou (smear)
PAR	postanesthetic recovery
p.c.	after meals
PCI	percutaneous coronary intervention
PD	panic disorder
PDA	patent ductus arteriosus
PE	physical examination; pulmonary embolism; polyethylene
PEFR	peak expiratory flow rate
per	by or through

BOX 8-1 Abbreviations Commonly Used in Documentation (*Cont.*)

Abbreviation or Symbol	Meaning
PERRLA	pupils equal, round, and reactive to light and accommodation
PET	positron emission tomography
PF	peak flow
PFT	pulmonary function testing
pH	potential of hydrogen
PH	past history
PI	present illness
PID	pelvic inflammatory disease
PIH	pregnancy-induced hypertension
p.m.	after noon
PLT	platelet
PMH	past medical history
PMN	polymorphonuclear (leukocyte)
PNS	peripheral nervous system
p.o.	by mouth
post-op or postop	postoperative
PPBS	postprandial blood sugar
PR	per rectum
pre-op or preop	preoperative
p.r.n. or prn	as needed
PSA	prostate-specific antigen
PSG	polysomnography
pt	patient
PT	physical therapy; prothrombin time
PTCA	percutaneous transluminal coronary angioplasty
PTH	parathyroid hormone
PTSD	posttraumatic stress disorder
PTT	partial thromboplastin time
PUD	peptic ulcer disease

BOX 8-1 Abbreviations Commonly Used in Documentation (*Cont.*)

Abbreviation or Symbol	Meaning
PV	per vagina
PVC	premature ventricular contraction
Px	physical examination
q	every
q.d.	every day, daily
qh	every hour
q2h	every 2 hours
q.i.d.	four times a day
q.o.d.	every other day
qt	quart
R	respiration
℞	right
RA	rheumatoid arthritis
RBC	red blood cell; red blood count
RLQ	right lower quadrant
R/O	rule out
ROM	range of motion
ROS	review of symptoms
RP	retrograde pyelogram
RRR	regular rate and rhythm
RTC	return to clinic
RTO	return to office
RUQ	right upper quadrant
Rx	recipe; prescription
s̄	without
S	subjective
SA	sinoatrial
SAB	spontaneous abortion
SAD	seasonal affective disorder
SC	subcutaneous
SCA	sudden cardiac arrest

BOX 8-1 Abbreviations Commonly Used in Documentation (*Cont.*)

Abbreviation or Symbol	Meaning
SCC	squamous cell carcinoma
SH	social history
Sig:	instruction to patient
SLE	systemic lupus erythematosus
SOB	shortness of breath
SPECT	single-photon emission computed tomography
SpGr	specific gravity
SQ	subcutaneous
SR	systems review
$\overline{\overline{ss}}$	one-half
STAT	immediately
STD	sexually transmitted disease
SUI	stress urinary incontinence
suppos	suppository
SV	stroke volume
Sx	symptom
T	temperature
T_3	triiodothyronine
T_4	thyroxine
T&A	tonsillectomy and adenoidectomy
tab	tablet
TAB	therapeutic abortion
TB	tuberculosis
TEDS	thromboembolic disease stockings
TEE	transesophageal echocardiogram
TIA	transient ischemic attack
t.i.d. or tid	three times a day
TM	tympanic membrane
TMR	transmyocardial revascularization
tPA or TPA	tissue plasminogen activator

BOX 8-1	Abbreviations Commonly Used in Documentation (*Cont.*)

Abbreviation or Symbol	Meaning
Tr	treatment
TSH	thyroid-stimulating hormone
TURP	transurethral resection of the prostate
TV	tidal volume
Tx	treatment; traction
UA	urinalysis
UCHD	usual childhood diseases
URI	upper respiratory infection
US or U/S	ultrasound
UTI	urinary tract infection
VC	vital capacity
VCU or VCUG	voiding cystourethrogram
V/Q	ventilation/perfusion
VS	vital signs
VSD	ventricular septal defect
V_T	tidal volume
w.a.	while awake
WBC	white blood cell; white blood count
WDWN	well developed, well nourished
wk	week
WNL	within normal limits
Wt	weight
x	times; for
x-ray	radiography
y.o. or y/o	year old
yr	year
♀	female
♂	male
#	number; pound
°	degree; hour
↑	increase; above

BOX 8-1	Abbreviations Commonly Used in Documentation (*Cont.*)
Abbreviation or Symbol	**Meaning**
↓	decrease; below
✓	check
∅	none; negative
♀ standing symbol	standing
sitting symbol	sitting
lying symbol	lying
×	times; for
>	greater than
<	less than
†	one
††	two
†††	three
†v	four
I, II, III, IV, V, VI, VII, VIII, IX, and **X**	uppercase Roman numerals 1–10

From Willis MC. *Medical Terminology: The Language of Health Care*, 2nd ed. Baltimore: Lippincott Williams & Wilkins, 2006.

BOX 8-2 Celsius–Fahrenheit Temperature Conversion Scale

Celsius to Fahrenheit

Use the following formula to convert Celsius readings to Farenheit readings:

$$°F = 9/5 \times °C + 32$$

For example, if the Celsius reading is 37°:

$$°F = (9/5 \times 37) + 32$$
$$= 66.6 + 32$$
$$= 98.6°F \text{ (normal body temperature)}$$

Fahrenheit to Celsius

Use the following formula to convert Fahrenheit readings to Celsius readings:

$$°C = 5/9(°F - 32)$$

For example, if the Fahrenheit reading is 68°:

$$°C = 5/9(68 - 32)$$
$$= 5/9 \times 36$$
$$= 20°C \text{ (a nice spring day)}$$

From Memmler RL, Cohen BJ, Wood, DL. *The Human Body in Health and Disease*, 10th ed. Baltimore: Lippincott Williams & Wilkins, 2005.

BOX 8-2 **Celsius–Fahrenheit Temperature Conversion Scale (*Cont.*)**

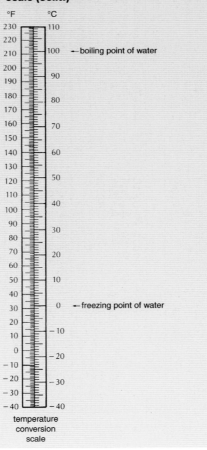

temperature
conversion
scale

TABLE 8-2	Metric Measurements		
Unit	**Abbreviation**	**Metric Equivalent**	**U.S. Equivalent**
Units of Length			
kilometer	km	1000 m	0.62 miles; 1.6 km/mile
meter*	m	100 cm; 1000 mm	39.4 inches; 1.1 yards
centimeter	cm	1/100 m; 0.01 m	0.39 inches; 2.5 cm/inch
millimeter	mm	1/1000 m; 0.001 m	0.039 inches; 25 mm/inch
micrometer	μm	1/1000 mm; 0.001 mm	
Units of Weight			
kilogram	kg	1000 g	2.2 lb
gram*	g	1000 mg	0.035 oz; 28.5 g/oz
milligram	mg	1/1000 g; 0.001 g	
microgram	μg, mcg	1/1000 mg; 0.001 mg	
Units of Volume			
liter*	L	1000 mL	1.06 qt
deciliter	dL	1/10 L; 0.1 L	
milliliter	mL	1/1000 L; 0.001 L	
microliter	μL	1/1000 mL; 0.001 mL	0.034 oz; 29.4 mL/oz

*Basic unit.

BOX 8-3 Key English to Spanish Health Care Phrases

Introductory Phrases

please	por favor	por fah-*vor*
thank you	gracias	*grah*-see-ahs
good morning	buenos días	*bway*-nos *dee*-ahs
good afternoon	buenas tárdes	*bway*-nas *tar*-days
good evening	buenas noches	*bway*-nas *noh*-chays
my name is	mi nombre es	me *nohm*-bray ays
yes/no	si/no	see/no
What is your name?	¿Cómo se llama?	¿Koh-moh say jah-mah?
How old are you?	¿Cuántos años tienes?	¿*Kwan*-tohs ahn-yos tee-*aynj*ays?
Do you understand me?	¿Me entiende?	¿Me ayn-tee-*ayn*-day?
How do you feel?	¿Cómo se siente?	¿*Koh*-moh say see-*ayn*-tay?
physician	médico	*may*-dee-koh
hospital	hospital	*ooh*-spee-tall

General

zero	cero	*se*-roh
one	uno	*oo*-noh
two	dos	dohs
three	tres	trays
four	cuatro	*kwah*-troh
five	cinco	*sin*-koh
six	seis	says
seven	siete	see-*ay*-tay
eight	ocho	oh-choh
nine	nueve	new-*ay*-vay
ten	diez	*dee*-ays

BOX 8-3 **Key English to Spanish Health Care Phrases (*Cont.*)**

Sunday	domingo	doh-*ming*-goh
Monday	lunes	*loo*-nays
Tuesday	martes	*mar*-tays
Wednesday	miércoles	mee-*er*-cohl-ays
Thursday	jueves	*hway*-vays
Friday	viernes	vee-*ayr*-nays
Saturday	sábado	*sah*-bah-doh
right	derecho	day-*ray*-choh
left	izqierdo	ees-kee-*ayr*-doh
in the daytime	en el dìa	ayn el *dee*-ah
at noon	a mediodía	ah meh-dee-oh-*dee*-ah
at bedtime	al acostarse	al ah-kos-*tar*-say
at night	por la noche	por la *noh*-chay
today	ñoy	oy
tomorrow	mañana	mah-*nyah*-nah
yesterday	ayer	ai-*yer*

Parts of the Body

the head	la cabeza	la kah-*bay*-sah
the eye	el ojo	el *o*-hoh
the ears	los oídos	lohs-o-*ee*-dohs
the nose	la nariz	la nah-*reez*
the mouth	la boca	lah *boh*-kah
the tongue	la lengua	la *len*-gwah
the neck	el cuello	el-koo-*eh*-joh
the throat	la garganta	lah gar-*gan*-tah
the skin	la piel	la pee-el
the bones	los huesos	lohs hoo-*ay*-sos
the muscles	los músculos	lohs *moos*-koo-lohs
the nerves	los nervios	lohs *nayhr*-vee-ohs

BOX 8-3 Key English to Spanish Health Care Phrases (*Cont.*)

the shoulder blades	las paletillas	lahs pah-lay-*tee*-jahs
the arm	el brazo	el *brah*-soh
the elbow	el codo	el *koh*-doh
the wrist	la muñeca	lah moon-*yeh*-kah
the hand	la mano	lah *mah*-noh
the chest	el pecho	el *pay*-choh
the lungs	los pulmones	lohs puhl-*moh*-nays
the heart	el corazón	el koh-rah-*son*
the ribs	las costillas	lahs kohs-*tee*-jahs
the side	el flanco	el *flahn*-koh
the back	la espalda	lay ays-*pahl*-dah
the abdomen	el abdomen	el ahb-*doh*-men
the stomach	el estómago	el ays-*toh*-mah-goh
the leg	la pierna	lah pee-ehr-nah
the thigh	el muslo	el *moos*-loh
the ankle	el tobillo	el toh-*bee*-joh
the foot	el pie	el *pee*-ay
urine	urino	u-*re*-noh

Examination

Remove your clothing.	Quítese su ropa.	*Key*-tay-say soo *roh*-pah.
Put on this gown.	Pongáse la bata.	Phon-*gah*-say lah *bah*-tah.
Be seated.	Siéntese.	See-*ayn*-tay-say.
Recline.	Acuestése.	Ah-*cways*-tay-say.
Sit up.	Siéntese.	See-*ayn*-tay-say
Stand.	Parése.	*Pah*-ray-say.
Bend your knees.	Doble las rodíllas.	*Doh*-blay lahs roh-*dee*-yahs.

BOX 8-3	Key English to Spanish Health Care Phrases (*Cont.*)	
Do not move.	No se muéva.	No say moo-*ay*-vah.
Turn on (or to) your left side.	Voltéese a su lado izquierdo.	Vohl-*tay*-sah ah soo *lah*-doh is-key-*ayr*-doh.
Turn on (or to) your right side.	Voltéese a su lado derecho.	Vohl-*tay*-say ah soo *lah*-doh day-*ray*-choh.
Take a deep breath.	Respíra profúndo.	Ray-*speer*-rah pro-*foon*-doh.
Treatment		
It is necessary.	Es nesesario.	Ays neh-say-*sah*-ree-oh.
a prescription	una receta	*oo*-na ray-say-tah
Use it regularly.	Tómelo con regularidad.	*Toh*-may-loh kohn ray-goo-*lay*-ree-dad.
before meals	antes des comidas	*ahn*-tays day lahs koh-*mee*-dahs
after meals	despues de las comidas	*days*-poo-ehs day lahs koh-*mee*-dahs
every day	todos los días	*toh*-dohs lohs *dee*-ah
every hour	cada hora	*kah*-dah *oh*-rah
General		
How do you feel?	¿Cómo se siénte?	¿*Koh*-moh say see-*ayn*-tay?
Do you have pain?	¿Tiéne dolor?	¿Tee-*ay*-nay doh-*lorh*?

BOX 8-3 Key English to Spanish Health Care Phrases (*Cont.*)

Where is the pain?	¿Adónde es el dolor?	¿Ah-*dohn*-day ays ayl doh-*lorh*?
You may not eat/drink.	No coma/béba.	Noh *koh*-mah/bay-*bah*.
I am going to . . .	Voy a . . .	Voy ah . . .
Count (take) your pulse.	Tomár su púlso.	Toh-*mahr* soo *pool*-soh.
Take your temperature.	Tomár su temperatúra.	Toh-*mahr* soo taym-pay-rah-*too*-rah.
Take your blood pressure.	Tomar su presión.	Toh-*mahr* soo pray-see-*ohn*.
Give you pain medicine.	Dárle medicación para dolor.	*Dahr*-lay may dee-kah-see-*ohn* pah-rah doh-*lohr*.
It is important to . . .	Es importánte que . . .	Ays eem-por-*tahn*-tay kay . . .
Walk (ambulate).	Caminar.	Kah-mee-*narh*.
Drink fluids.	Beber líquidos.	Bay-*bayr lee*-kay-dohs.
Have you had anything to eat or drink since midnight last night?	¿Comió o bebió ustedalgo después de la medianoche?	

BOX 8-4 Commonly Misused Words

adverse (harmful)
averse (opposed to)

affect (verb, to influence, change)
effect (noun, result)

already (previously)
all ready (prepared, all set)

anoxia (without oxygen)
anorexia (without appetite)

aphagia (without swallowing)
aphasia (without speech)

appendices (end of book)
appendicitis (inflammation of
  appendix)

biannual (twice a year)
biennial (occurring every 2 years)

bite (grip with teeth)
byte (character)

bowl (container)
bowel (intestines, colon)

emphysema (chronic lung
  disease)
empyema (accumulation of pus)

ensure (be certain)
insure (protect against risk)
assure (provide confidence)

everyday (adjective, routine,
  ordinary)
every day (adverbial phrase,
  each day)

except (exclude)
expect (anticipate)
accept (agree)

farther (greater distance)
further (greater degree)

fundus (pertains to hollow
  organ)
fungus (organism that can lead
  to infection)

its (possessive pronoun)
it's (contraction of it and is)

lactose (type of sugar in
  milk)
lactase (enzyme)

libel (written defamatory
  statement)
liable (legally responsible)

may be (compound verb)
maybe (adverb, perhaps)

metatarsals (bones in foot)
metacarpals (bones in palm)

BOX 8-4 Commonly Misused Words (*Cont.*)

mucus (substance that is secreted)
mucous (membrane that secretes)

parental (pertaining to parent)
parenteral (not by mouth)

postnatal (after birth)
postnasal (behind nose)

principle (noun, law)
principal (noun, leader; adjective, most important)

rubella (German measles)
rubeola (14-day measles)

serum (watery component of blood)
sebum (oily substance secreted by the sebaceous glands)

tact (behavior)
tack (different direction)

than (to show comparison)
then (next)

there (place, point)
their (possessive pronoun)
they're (pronoun plus verb)

uvula (soft tissue at back of palate)
vulva (external female organ)

weather (climate)
whether (indicating a possibility)

TABLE 8-3 Word Parts and Their Meanings

Word Part	Meaning	Word Part	Meaning
a-	not, without, lack of, absence	amyl/o	starch
ab-	away from	an-	not, without, lack of, absence
abdomin/o	abdomen	andr/o	male
-ac	pertaining to	angi/o	vessel
acous, acus	sound, hearing	an/o	anus
acro-	extremity, end	ante-	before
ad-	toward, near	anti-	against
aden/o	gland	aort/o	aorta
adip/o	fat	-ar	pertaining to
adren/o	adrenal gland, epinephrine	arter/o, arteri/o	artery
adrenal/o	adrenal gland	arteriol/o	arteriole
adrenocortic/o	adrenal cortex	anthr/o	joint
-al	air, gas	-ary	pertaining to
alg/o, algi/o, algesi/o	pain	-ase	enzyme
-algesia	pain	atel/o	incomplete
-algia	pain	atlant/o	atlas
ambly-	dim	atri/o	atrium
amnio	amnion	audi/o	hearing
		auto-	self

TABLE 8-3 Word Parts and Their Meanings (Continued)

Word Part	Meaning	Word Part	Meaning
azo, azot/o	nitrogenous compounds	calc/i	calcium
		cali/o, calic/o	calyx
		-capnia	carbon dioxide (level of)
bacill/i, bacill/o	bacillus	carcin/o	cancer, carcinoma
bacteri/o	bacterium	cardi/o	heart
balan/o	glans penis	cec/o	cecum
bi-	two, twice	-cele	hernia, localized dilation
bili	bile		
blast/o, -blast	immature cell, productive cell, embryonic cell	celi/o	abdomen
		centesis	puncture, tap
		cephal/o	head
blephar/o	eyelid	cerebell/o	cerebellum
brachi/o	arm	cerebr/o	cerebrum
brachy-	short	cervic/o	neck, cervix
brady-	slow	chem/o	chemical
bronch/o, bronch/l	bronchus	cheil/o	lip
bronchiol	bronchiole	cholangi/o	bile duct
bucc/o	cheek	chol/e, chol/o	bile, gall
burs/o	bursa		

TABLE 8-3 Word Parts and Their Meanings (Continued)

Word Part	Meaning	Word Part	Meaning
cholecyst/o	gallbladder	crani/o	skull, cranium
choledoch/o	common bile duct	cry/o	cold
chondr/o	cartilage	crypt/o	hidden
chori/o, choroid/o	choroid	-cus	sound, hearing
chrom/o, chromat/o	color, stain	cyan/o	blue
chron/o	time	cycl/o	ciliary body, ciliary muscle (of eye)
circum-	around		
clasis, -clasia	breaking	cyst/o, cyst/i	cyst, bladder, filled sac or pouch, urinary bladder
clitor/o, clitorid/o	clitoris		
coccy, coccyg/o	coccyx		
cochle/o	cochlea (of inner ear)	-cyte, cyt/o	cell
col/o, colon/o	colon		
colp/o	vagina	dacry/o	tear, lacrimal
contra-	against, opposite		apparatus
copro	feces	dacryocyst/o	lacrimal sac
corne/o	cornea	dactyl/o	finger, toe
cortic/o	outer portion, cerebral cortex	de-	down, without, removal, loss
cost/o	rib	dent/o, dent/i	tooth, teeth
counter-	opposite, against	derm/o, dermat/o	skin

TABLE 8-3 Word Parts and Their Meanings (*Continued*)

Word Part	Meaning	Word Part	Meaning
-desis	binding, fusion	electr/o	electricity
dextr/o-	right	embry/o	embryo
di-	two, twice	-emesis	vomiting
dia-	through	-emia	condition of blood
dilation, dilatation	expansion, widening	encephal/o	brain
dipl/o-o	double	end/o-	in, within
dis-	absence, removal, separation	endocrin/o	endocrine
		enter/o	intestine
duoden/o	duodenum	epi-	on, over
dys-	abnormal, painful, difficult	epididym/o	epididymis
		episi/o	vulva
		equi-	equal, same
ec-	out, outside	erg/o	work
ectasia, ectasis	dilation, dilatation, distension	erythr/o-	red, red blood cell
		erythrocyte/o	red blood cell
ecto-	out, outside	esophag/o	esophagus
-ectomy	excision, surgical removal	-esthesia, -esthesi/o	sensation
		eu-	true, good, easy, normal
edema	accumulation of fluid, swelling	ex/o-	away from, outside

251

TABLE 8-3 Word Parts and Their Meanings (Continued)

Word Part	Meaning	Word Part	Meaning
extra-	outside	glyc/o	sugar, glucose
		gnath/o	jaw
fasci/o	fascia	goni/o	angle
fer	to carry	-gram	record of data
ferr/i, ferr/o	iron	-graph	instrument for recording data
fet/o	fetus		
fibr/o	fiber	-graphy	act of recording data
-form	like, resembling		
		gravida	pregnant woman
galact/o	milk	gyn/o, gynec/o	woman
gangli/o, ganglion/o	ganglion		
gastr/o	stomach	hem/o, hemat/o	blood
gen, genesis	origin, formation	hemi-	half, one side
ger/e, ger/o	old age	-hernia	condition of blood
-geusia	sense of taste	hepat/o	liver
gingiv/o	gum, gingiva	hetero-	other, different,
gli/o	neuroglia		unequal
glomerul/o	glomerulus	hidr/o	sweat, perspiration
gloss/o	tongue	hist/o, histi/o	tissue
gluc/o	glucose	homo-, homeo-	same, unchanging

TABLE 8-3 Word Parts and Their Meanings (Continued)

Word Part	Meaning	Word Part	Meaning
hydr/o	water, fluid	-ics	medical specialty
hyper-	over, excess, increased, abnormally high	-ile	pertaining to
		ile/o	ileum
		ili/o	ilium
hypn/o	sleep	im-	not
hypo-	under, below, decreased, abnormally low	immun/o	immunity, immune system
		in-	not
hypophys	pituitary, hypophysis	infra-	below
hyster/o	uterus	in/o	fiber, muscle fiber
		insul/o	pancreatic islets
-ia	condition of	inter-	between
-ian	specialist	intra-	in, within
-is/sis	condition of	ir, irit/o, irid/o	iris
-iatrics	medical specialty	-ism	condition of
-iatr/o	physician	iso-	equal, same
-iatry	medical specialty	-ist	specialist
-ic	pertaining to	-itis	inflammation
-ical	pertaining to	jejun/o	jejunum

253

TABLE 8-3 Word Parts and Their Meanings (Continued)

Word Part	Meaning	Word Part	Meaning
juxta-	near, beside	-lepsy	seizure
		leuk/o-	white, colorless,
kali	potassium		white blood cell
kary/o	nucleus	leukocyt/o	white blood cell
kerat/o	cornea, keratin,	-lexia	reading
	horny layer of skin	lingu/o	tongue
kin/o, kine, kinesi/o,	movement	lip/o	fat, lipid
kinet/o		-listhesis	slipping
		lith	calculus, stone
labi/o	lip	-logy	study of
labyrinth/o	labyrinth (inner ear)	lumb/o	lumbar region, lower
lacrim/o	tear, lacrimal		back
	apparatus	lymphaden/o	lymph node
lact/o	milk	lymphangi/o	lymphatic vessel
-lalia	speech, babble	lymph/o	lymph, lymphatic
lapar/o	abdominal wall		system,
laryng/o	larynx		lymphocyte
lenti	lens	lymphocyt/o	lymphocyte

TABLE 8-3	Word Parts and Their Meanings (Continued)		
Word Part	Meaning	Word Part	Meaning
-lysis	separation, loosening, dissolving, destruction		oblongata, spinal cord
		mega-, megalo-	large, abnormally large
-lytic	dissolving, reducing, loosening	-megaly	enlargement
		melan/o-	black, dark, melanin
		mening/o, meninge/o	meninges
macro-	large, abnormally large	men/o, mens	month, menstruation
mal-	bad, poor	mes/o-	middle
malacia	softening	-meter	instrument for measuring
mamm/o	breast, mammary gland	metr/o	measure
-mania	excited state, obsession	metr/o, metr/l	uterus
		-metry	measurement of
mast/o	breast, mammary gland	micro-	small, one millionth
medull/o	inner part, medulla	-mimetic	mimicking, simulating

TABLE 8-3	Word Parts and Their Meanings (Continued)		
Word Part	**Meaning**	**Word Part**	**Meaning**
mon/o	one	nephr/o	kidney
morph/o	form, structure	neur/o, neur/l	nervous system, nerve
muc/o	mucus, mucous membrane	noct/l	night
multi-	many	non-	not
muscul/o	muscle	normo-	normal
myc/o	fungus, mold	nucle/o	nucleus
myel/o	bone marrow, spinal cord	nyct/o	night, darkness
my/o	muscle	ocul/o	eye
myring/o	tympanic membrane	odont/o	tooth, teeth
myx/o	mucus	-odynia	pain
narc/o	stupor, unconsciousness	-oid	like, resembling
nas/o	nose	olig/o-	few, scanty, deficiency of
nat/i	birth	-ome	tumor
natri	sodium	onc/o	tumor
necrosis	death of tissue	onych/o	nail
neo-	new	oo	ovum
		oophor/o	ovary

TABLE 8-3 Word Parts and Their Meanings *(Continued)*

Word Part	Meaning	Word Part	Meaning
ophthalm/o	eye	ox/y	oxygen, sharp, acute
-opia	eye, vision		
-opsia	vision		
opt/o	eye, vision	pachy-	thick
orchid/o, orchi/o	testis	palat/o	palate
or/o	mouth	palpebr/o	eyelid
ortho-	straight, correct, upright	pan-	all
		pancreat/o	pancreas
-ory	pertaining to	papill/o	nipple
osche/o	scrotum	para-	near, beside, abnormal
-ose	sugar		
-o/sis	condition of	para	woman who has given birth
-osmia	sense of smell	parathyr/o,	parathyroid
oste/o	bone	parathyroid/o	
ot/o	ear	-paresis	partial paralysis
-ous	pertaining to	-path/o, -pathy	disease, any disease of
ovari/o	ovary		
ov/o, ovul/o	ovum	ped/o	foot, child
-oxia	oxygen (level of)		

257

TABLE 8-3 Word Parts and Their Meanings (Continued)

Word Part	Meaning	Word Part	Meaning
pelvi/o	pelvis	phrenic/o	phrenic nerve
-penia	decrease in, deficiency of	phyt/o	plant
per-	through	pituitar	pituitary, hypophysis
peri-	around	plas, -plasia	formation, molding, development
perine/o	perineum	-plasty	plastic repair, plastic surgery, reconstruction
periton, peritone/o	peritoneum		
-pexy	surgical fixation	-plegia	paralysis
phac/o, phak/o	lens	pleur/o	pleura
phag/o	eat, ingest	-pnea	breathing
pharm, pharmac/o	drug, medicine	pneum/o, pneumat/o	air, gas, lung, respiration
pharyng/o	pharynx		
-phasia	speech	pneumon/o	lung
phil, -philic	attracting, absorbing	pod/o	foot
phleb/o	vein	-poiesis	formation, production
-phobia	fear	poikilo-	varied, irregular
phon/o	sound, voice	poly-	many, much
-phonia	voice	post-	after, behind
phot/o	light		
phren/o	diaphragm		

TABLE 8-3 Word Parts and Their Meanings (Continued)

Word Part	Meaning	Word Part	Meaning
pre-	before, in front of	quadr/i	four
presby-	old		
prim/i-	first	rachi/o	spine
pro-	before, in front of	radicul/o	root of spinal nerve
proct/o	rectum	radi/o	radiation, x-ray
prostat/o	prostate	re-	again, back
prote/o	protein	rect/o	rectum
pseudo-	false	ren/o	kidney
psych/o	mind	reticul/o	network
ptosis	dropping, downward displacement, prolapse	retin/o	retina
		retro-	behind, backward
		rhabd/o	rod, muscle cell
ptysis	spitting	-rhage, -rhagia	bursting forth, profuse flow,
puer	child		hemorrhage
pulm/o, pulmon/o	lung	-rhaphy	surgical repair, suture
pupill/o	pupil		
pyel/o	renal pelvis	-rhea	flow, discharge
pylor/o	pylorus	-rhexis	rupture
py/o	pus	rhin/o	nose
pyr/o, pyret/o	fever, fire		

TABLE 8-3 Word Parts and Their Meanings *(Continued)*

Word Part	Meaning	Word Part	Meaning
sacchar/o	sugar	sial/o	saliva, salivary gland, salivary duct
sacr/o	sacrum	sider/o	iron
salping/o	tube, oviduct, eustachian (auditory) tube	sigmoid/o	sigmoid colon
		sinistr/o	left
-schisis	fissure, splitting	-sis	condition of
scler/o	hard, sclera (of eye)	somat/o	body
sclerosis	hardening	-some	body, small body
-scope	instrument for viewing or examining	somn/i, somn/o	sleep
		son/o	sound, ultrasound
-scopy	examination of	spasm	sudden contraction, cramp
seb/o	sebum, sebaceous gland	sperm/i	semen, spermatozoa
semi-	half, partial	spermat/o	semen, spermatozoa
semin	semen	-spermia	condition of semen
sept/o	septum, dividing wall, partition	spir/o	breathing
		splen/o	spleen

TABLE 8-3 Word Parts and Their Meanings (Continued)			
Word Part	Meaning	Word Part	Meaning
spondyl/o	vertebra	synovi/i	synovial joint, synovial member
staped/o, stapedi/o	stapes		
staphyl/o	grapelike cluster, staphylococcus		
		tachy-	rapid
stasis	suppression, stoppage	tax/o	order, arrangement
		tel/e-, tel/o-	end
steat/o	fatty	ten/o, tendin/o	tendon
stenosis	narrowing, constriction	terat/o	malformed fetus
		test/o	testis, testicle
		tetra-	four
steth/o	chest	thalam/o	thalamus
sthen/o	strength	therm/o	heat, temperature
stoma, stomat/o	mouth	thorac/o	chest, thorax
-stomy	surgical creation of an opening	thromb/o	blood clot
		thrombocyt/o	platelet, thrombocyte
strept/o-	twisted chain, strepto coccus	thym/o	thymus gland
		thyr/o, thyroid/o	thyroid
sub-	below, under	toc/o	labor
super-	above, excess	-tome	instrument for incising
supra-	above		
syn-, sym-	together		

TABLE 8-3 Word Parts and Their Meanings *(Continued)*

Word Part	Meaning	Word Part	Meaning
-tomy	incision, cutting	un-	not
ton/o	tone	uni-	one
tonsill/o	tonsil	-uresis	urination
tox/o, toxic/o	poison, toxin	ureter/o	ureter
toxin	poison	urethr/o	urethra
trache/o	trachea	-uria	condition of urine, urination
trans-	through	ur/o	urine, urinary tract
tri-	three	urin/o	urine
trich/o	hair	uter/o	uterus
-tripsy	crushing	uve/o	uvea (of eye)
trop-, -tropic	act(ing) on, affecting	uvul/o	uvula
troph/o, -trophy	feeding, growth, nourishment	vagin/o	sheath, vagina
-trophia		valv/o, valvul/o	valve
tympan/o	tympanic cavity (middle ear), tympanic membrane	varic/o	twisted and swollen vein, varix
		vascul/o	vessel

TABLE 8-3	Word Parts and Their Meanings (Continued)		
Word Part	**Meaning**	**Word Part**	**Meaning**
vas/o deferens	vessel, duct, vas	vir/o	apparatus (of ear) virus
ven/o, ven/i	vein	vulv/o	vulva
ventricul/o	cavity, ventricle	xanth/o-	yellow
verterbr/o	vertebra, spinal column	xen/o xero-	foreign, strange dry
vesic/o	urinary bladder	-y	condition of
vesicul/o	seminal vesicle		
vestibul/o	vestibule, vestibular		

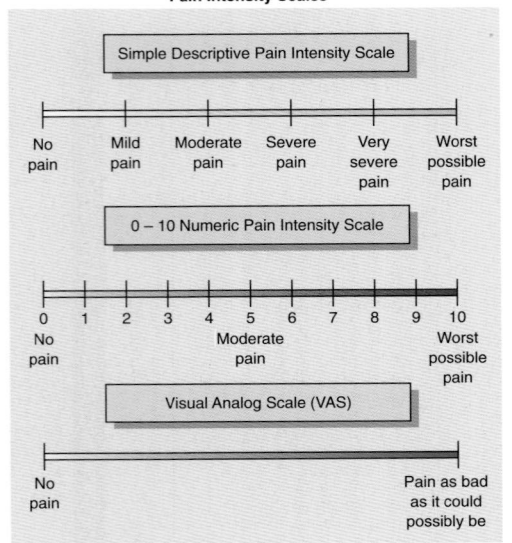

A 10-cm baseline is recommended for each of these scales.
Figure 8-2. Pain intensity scales.

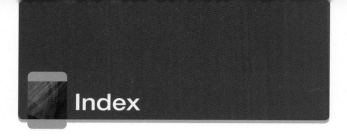

Index

Page numbers in *italics* denote figures; those followed by a t denote tables.